OXFORD MEDICAL PUBLICATIONS

Medical Research with Children: Ethics, Law, and Practice

Medical Research with Children: Ethics, Law, and Practice

*The report of an Institute of Medical Ethics
working group on the ethics of clinical
research investigations on children*

Edited by

RICHARD H. NICHOLSON, MA, BM, DCH

Deputy Director, Institute of Medical Ethics

OXFORD NEW YORK TOKYO
OXFORD UNIVERSITY PRESS · 1986

Oxford University Press, Walton Street, Oxford OX2 6DP

Oxford New York Toronto
Delhi Bombay Calcutta Madras Karachi
Kuala Lumpur Singapore Hong Kong Tokyo
Nairobi Dar es Salaam Cape Town
Melbourne Auckland
and associated companies in
Beirut Berlin Ibadan Nicosia

Published in the United States
by Oxford University Press, New York

British Library Cataloguing in Publication Data

Medical research with children: ethics, law and practice: the report of an Institute of
Medical Ethics Working group on the ethics of clinical research investigations on
children. — (Oxford medical publications)
1. Human experimentation in medicine   2. Pediatrics — Research   3. Medical
ethics
I. Nicholson, Richard H.   II. Institute of Medical Ethics
174'.28   R853.H8
ISBN 0–19–261528–9

Library of Congress Cataloging in Publication Data
Main entry under title:
Medical research with children.
(Oxford medical publications)
Includes bibliographies and index.
1. Pediatrics — Moral and ethical aspects.   2. Human experimentation in medicine
— Moral and ethical aspects.
I. Nicholson, Richard H.   II. Institute of Medical Ethics (Great Britain)
III. Series.   [DNLM: 1. Ethics, Medical.   2. Human Experimentation — in
infancy & childhood.   3. Informed Consent.   4. Research. WS 20 M489]
RJ47.M435   1985   174'.28   85-31030
ISBN 0–19–261528–9

Set by Northumberland Press, Gateshead
Printed in Great Britain by
Richard Clay (The Chaucer Press) Ltd,
Bungay, Suffolk

Foreword

It is right that the restless human mind should pause from time to time to scrutinize its own pursuits. In our lifetime the art of medicine has been grounded anew in medical science, much of it the product of systematic research — a process extended and accelerated, probably, more in the last half century than in any age before. Throughout this period an anxiety about the aims, scope, methods, and costs of research has never been far away. It expressed itself, in revulsion from the Nazi atrocities, in the Code of Nuremberg and then in a series of Declarations from the World Medical Association. To these have been added codes of practice and institutional safeguards by national and professional bodies.

The anxiety shows no sign of lessening. It is particularly evident over paediatric research, because children are so vulnerable and have a special claim to protection, by their parents first, and then by the community as a whole in conventions and laws. As guidelines for research involving children multiplied, so did inconsistencies in their prescriptions. It was suggested to the Society for the Study of Medical Ethics (now the Institute of Medical Ethics) that it might usefully study the question afresh and publish a Report designed to encourage reflection and, perhaps, to help members of Research Ethics Committees in the discharge of their duties. The Leverhulme Trust provided funds for the exercise, and thanks are due to the Trustees for their generous grant.

A Group was convened, with practitioners balanced by others representing relevant disciplines and interests. The names of members are printed on another page. It met twenty-five times over three years, to discuss prepared papers. It sought the material for its study in the literature, in reported practice, and by means of an enquiry sent to all the identifiable Research Ethics Committees in England and Wales. Two chapters in the Report derive, properly, from the philosophers and lawyers respectively in the Group. The others are the work of our Research Fellow, Dr R. H. Nicholson, who knows now (if he knew not before) what it is to be under the concentrated scrutiny of thirty-six critical eyes and to have survived with respect and affection unimpaired.

It is the task of the Chairman, on his own behalf and on that of the Institute of Medical Ethics, to express thanks to members, and especially to Dr Nicholson, for their unswerving application of themselves to the task; to the Chairmen of those Research Ethics Committees who replied to our enquiry; to individuals who gave us personal evidence, notably Professor Spyros Doxiadis, of the Foundation for Research in Childhood in Athens, and Miss Mary Dunne, Director of Nursing at the Portland Hospital, London; and to the Director and Staff of the Ciba Foundation for the hospitality and conference facilities of their House, where all our meetings were held.

Before we could complete our discussions we were saddened by the death of Mrs Mia Kellmer Pringle. From her place, next but one to the right of the Chair, had come always at the right moment, quiet but apt and penetrating interventions, potent in their brevity, whenever some true interest of the child seemed to be in question. She embodied not simply a concern for children but an effective concern, with an intellect skilled to search out the means to assure the end which mind and heart alike required.

We hope that our Report will help its readers in their planning and oversight of research, so properly conducted as to serve the common interest of children in health and in sickness without invading the interest of any single child.

G. R. DUNSTAN
Chairman

Contents

Acknowledgements

The editor is very grateful for permission from Sir Edward Pochin to reprint, with slight amendments, the material in Tables 5.1–5.4, and from Professor Rachel Rosser to reprint the material in Table 5.5.

In developing the questionnaire, used in the survey of research ethics committees reported in Chapter 8, the editor was assisted not only by members of the working group, but also by very useful discussions with two senior research officers at the National Children's Bureau: Ann Bowling and Peter Shepherd. Analysis of the survey results would not have been possible without the considerable help of two members of the working group, Brendan Callaghan and David Hall.

Finally, the editor would like to thank Pauline Bunting for her very accurate typing of the manuscript, and the staff of Oxford University Press for all their help in seeing the report through to its published form.

Members of the working group

Professor G. R. Dunstan, M.A., D.D., F.S.A., (Chairman)
Emeritus Professor of Moral and Social Theology in the University of London. Honorary Research Fellow in the University of Exeter.

Mrs Priscilla Alderson, B.A.
Former chairman of the National Association for the Welfare of Children in Hospital.

Dr Martin Brueton, M.D., M.Sc., M.R.C.P., D.C.H.
Senior Lecturer in Child Health, Charing Cross and Westminster Medical School, University of London. Honorary Consultant Paediatrician, Westminster Children's, St Stephen's, and Brompton Hospitals.

The Revd Brendan Callaghan, S.J., M.A., M.Phil., M.Th.
Principal, Heythrop College, University of London.

Professor Gerald Dworkin, LL.B.
Professor of Law, University of Southampton.

Dr Raanan Gillon, B.A., M.B., B.S., M.R.C.P.
Editor, *Journal of Medical Ethics*; Director, College Health Service, Imperial College, University of London.

Professor Philip Graham, F.R.C.P., F.R.C.Psych.
Walker Professor of Child Psychiatry, Institute of Child Health, London.

Dr David Hall, M.A., M.A.(Econ), Ph.D.
Lecturer in Sociology, University of Liverpool.

Professor Richard Hare, M.A., F.B.A.
Formerly White's Professor of Moral Philosophy, University of Oxford.

Professor Ian Kennedy, LL.M.
Professor of Medical Law and Ethics, King's College, University of London.

The Countess of Limerick, M.A.
Executive Vice-Chairman, Foundation for the Study of Infant Deaths.

Professor Thomas Oppé, C.B.E., M.B., F.R.C.P., D.C.H.
Professor of Paediatrics, St Mary's Hospital Medical School, University of London.

Dr Ruth Porter, F.R.C.P., F.R.C.Psych., D.C.H.
Formerly Deputy Director, The Ciba Foundation; Psychotherapist.

†Dr Mia Kellmer Pringle, C.B.E., Ph.D., D.Sc., F.B.Ps.S.
Founder, and former director, of the National Children's Bureau, London.

Mrs Claire Rayner, S.R.N.
Journalist and author; formerly paediatric departmental sister.

Dr Elliot Shinebourne, M.D., F.R.C.P.
Consultant Paediatric Cardiologist, Brompton Hospital; Senior Lecturer in Paediatrics, Cardiothoracic Institute, University of London.

Prebendary Edward Shotter, B.A.
Director, Institute of Medical Ethics.

Professor Lewis Spitz, M.B., ChB., Ph.D., F.R.C.S., F.R.C.S.E.
Nuffield Professor of Paediatric Surgery, Institute of Child Health; Honorary Consultant Paediatric Surgeon, Hospital for Sick Children, Great Ormond Street, London.

Dr Richard Nicholson, M.A., B.M., D.C.H., (Research Fellow)
Deputy Director, Institute of Medical Ethics.

1

Introduction

A few years ago there was concern in a London teaching hospital at the incidence of pneumonia in new-born infants caused by aspiration of meconium. When a fetus, in late pregnancy or during delivery, is subjected to greater than normal stress, it frequently passes the contents of its rectum, known as meconium, into the surrounding fluid, or liquor; when the new-born infant takes its first breath it may inhale some of the meconium-stained liquor, which will have been in its mouth and throat. This causes a reactive pneumonia, which can make the infant very ill, and can even be fatal. It was therefore proposed, at the teaching hospital, that an experimental study should be carried out to see whether one could wash out the meconium before it caused pneumonia. If meconium was seen to be in the infant's larynx, and was likely therefore also to have entered further into the lungs, attempts were made immediately to wash it out. This required a salt solution, saline, to be squirted into the infant's trachea and then sucked out again, taking with it any meconium that might have reached the lungs, while the infant's chest was firmly held by an assistant to prevent it from taking its first breath.

Such an experiment raises a number of problems of the sort that are discussed in this report. Normally, new drugs and therapies are tried out on animals before humans, yet it was difficult to find an animal model for meconium aspiration. The experiment seems a fairly simple way of trying to prevent a potentially life-threatening condition, yet one may predict possible dangers arising from it. The infant may gasp during the procedure so that both saline and meconium are carried well into the lungs, causing the problem which the experiment was designed to prevent, and adding to the amount of fluid which the infant has to clear from its lungs when it starts breathing. One is also delaying the start of breathing in an infant who has no other oxygen supply, without which brain damage might follow if ventilation is not established within a very few minutes. It is normal practice in medicine for consent to be obtained before any therapeutic intervention is carried out, and most guidelines for the conduct of research on human beings stress that voluntary informed consent is required before research procedures are performed. Yet the infant is obviously incapable of giving any sort of consent, and his parents are not asked, since the procedure must be carried out at a moment's notice if it is to have the best chance of success. The proposal to carry out this research was approved by a research ethics committee, and it has been suggested that that was an adequate safeguard for the parents and their infants, although such a suggestion might be rejected by both lawyers and other observers.

In fact, after the experimental procedure had been tried on a few infants it was abandoned, since it was found to cause more problems for the infants than it solved. A report of the project has never been published, so there is no guarantee that other teams of paediatricians may not try it again elsewhere.

Most clinical research on children does not raise problems of such difficulty as those in the above example. The procedures involved are usually much less risky, and are often entirely non-invasive; but even then there may be difficulties about whether or not it is necessary to ask for parental consent, for instance, or whether the research is legal if it is of no potential benefit to the child subject. That there should be such problems is obviously inherent in the nature of the activity of research on children; but attempts at resolution of the problems are hindered by the imprecision of controls over experiments on human beings and conflict between the various guidelines now current. The guidelines produced so far in the United Kingdom are those of the Medical Research Council,[1] the Royal College of Physicians,[2] the Department of Health and Social Security,[3] and the British Paediatric Association.[4] There are in addition the Helsinki Declaration[5] of the World Medical Association that is widely accepted internationally, and the Proposed International Guidelines[6] drawn up by the World Health Organisation and the Council for International Organisations of Medical Sciences which are under consideration at present. The most detailed previous assessment of the ethics of research on children was provided by the US National Commission for the Protection of Human Subjects of Biomedical and Behavioral Research in its Report and Recommendations.[7]

Control of experiments on human beings

Until recently, clinical investigation of a human subject was an activity that was controlled only by the nature of the relationship between the research worker and the subject of the experiments. The process therefore depended on the good faith of the investigator and the tolerance of the patient. When, however, public attention was drawn to the fact that some clinical investigations appeared to exploit, to put in hazard or to violate the subject, it was accepted that a measure of public involvement was required.

The first time that many people outside the medical profession became aware that medical experiments that violated subjects had taken place was during the Nuremberg Military Tribunals in 1946. Evidence was given that up to two hundred German doctors, some professors included, had performed criminal experiments, often with fatal outcome, on both prisoners-of-war and civilians.

Public interest in the surveillance of medical experiments was renewed in 1962 following the thalidomide disaster, which produced demands in many countries for better controls on the ways in which new drugs were tested and introduced into human therapy. During that time, the Medical Research Council, in its annual report for 1962–3, made a statement entitled 'Responsibility in investigations on human subjects'[1] that addressed some of the legal and ethical problems of clinical research. The World Medical Association, also recognizing the extremely rapid growth then occurring in the field of medical research, adopted in 1964 the 'Declaration of Helsinki: Recommendations guiding medical doctors in biomedical research involving human subjects'. (It was revised in 1975 and 1983.)[5]

In 1966, Henry Beecher, Professor of Research in Anaesthesia at the Harvard Medical School, published an article 'Ethics and clinical research'[8] in the *New England Journal of Medicine*; it was to be far-reaching in its effects. He drew attention to twenty-two reports of unethical clinical research, illustrating a variety of ethical problems, and in most of which patients had been put at considerable risk. Shortly before, the Surgeon-General of the United States had issued the first rule requiring institutions accepting federal funds to establish independent review of research projects before they were started.

The following year, 1967, saw the publication of the first report of the Royal College of Physicians 'Committee on the supervision of the ethics of clinical investigations in institutions', which also recommended that every hospital or institution in which clinical research was undertaken should have a group of doctors that 'should satisfy itself of the ethics of all proposed investigations'. In the same year, M. H. Pappworth published his book *Human guinea pigs*,[9] which detailed several hundred reports of medical experiments that he considered unethical, most of which had been carried out either in the United Kingdom or in the United States of America. He proposed that 'research committees', each with at least one lay member, should be established in every region to review the ethics of proposed investigations, and that, by law, they should be responsible to the General Medical Council.

Over the next few years many hospitals in the United Kingdom did establish ethics committees to review proposed clinical research investigations. Even to this day, however, there is no statutory duty on health authorities, boards of governors, or other hospital managers to set up such research ethics committees and, indeed, some have not yet done so. At the request of the Chief Medical Officer of the Department of Health and Social Security (DHSS) in 1973, the Royal College of Physicians committee again made recommendations,[2] suggesting principally (1) that all proposals for clinical research investigations should be referred to the appropriate ethics committee for approval, and (2) that there should be a lay member on each research ethics committee. The DHSS finally published an advisory circular in 1975[3] confirming the 1967 and 1973 recommendations of the Royal College of Physicians, but without giving them the force of statute.

The history of ethical review of medical research both in the United Kingdom and elsewhere is considered further in Chapter 8, in which are also recorded the results of a survey examining the present role and constitution of research ethics committees in England and Wales.

Guidelines for the conduct of research

Research ethics committees provide, more or less effectively, peer review of proposals for clinical research. In general, however, restraints on clinical research derive from the law and from what is acceptable to public opinion; neither of these approaches necessarily takes fully into account the moral aspect. The problems are particularly difficult in the case of children, because of the special status which they have in regard to both the law and public opinion. This has resulted in the publication of the four sets of guidelines, mentioned above, for the conduct of clinical research on children in the United Kingdom, all of which have been based on uncertain interpretations of the law, and none of which has provided any details about the moral basis for the guidelines which it offers.

There is still a fond belief amongst large sections of the general public that doctors have all taken the Hippocratic Oath before they may be allowed to practise. Even where this was the tradition, however, this habit has been dying out since the time of the Second World War, so that some doctors now have never even read the Oath. Much of the Oath remains relevant to the conduct of modern medicine, but it contains no specific mention of experiments, the medical practice of Hippocrates' day being based largely on observation and hypothesis rather than on scientific research. Nevertheless, two sentences of the Oath contain general injunctions that could be taken to cover the conduct of clinical research: 'I will use treatment to help the sick according to my ability and judgment, but never with a view to injury and wrong-doing'; and 'I will abstain from all intentional wrong-doing and harm, especially from abusing the bodies of man or woman, bond or free.'[10]

The great French physiologist, Claude Bernard, has often been called the father of modern clinical investigation; he was a powerful advocate of the need for experiments on man in order to advance understanding in both physiology and clinical medicine. He realized also, however, that there were limits to what might be done in experiments, as the following excerpt from *An introduction to the study of experimental medicine* published in 1865 indicates: 'The principle of medical and surgical morality, therefore, consists in never performing on man an experiment which might be harmful to him to any extent, even though the result might be highly advantageous to science, i.e. to the health of others. But performing experiments and operations exclusively from the point of view of the patient's own advantage does not prevent their turning out profitably to science.'[11]

The first guidelines for the conduct of research on humans that treated separately the problems of research on children were produced – somewhat surprisingly in view of subsequent events – by the German Ministry of the Interior in 1931.[12] The guidelines as a whole laid down many of the requirements for the ethical conduct of clinical research that are to be found in modern guidelines such as the Helsinki Declaration. Thus, they affirmed the experimenter's primary duty to his subject, the need always to obtain informed consent, the need to try out new treatments on animals before trying them on humans, and the need for results to be published accurately. The guidelines contain two statements about children: 'Application of a new treatment must be considered particularly carefully if it involves infants or adolescents of less than 18 years', and 'Experimentation on infants or persons of less than 18 years is forbidden even if it will only expose them to a very slight danger'. 'Experimentation' was defined as any intervention that did not contribute directly to the treatment of a particular case.

Such a prohibition of experiments on children was repeated by subsequent guidelines. The Judgement of the Nuremberg Military Tribunal in 1947 on several Nazi doctors, now known as the Nuremberg Code,[13] makes no particular reference to children, but states plainly that 'The voluntary consent of the human subject is absolutely essential', thus effectively precluding much research on children. The first statement on the subject in the United Kingdom was made by the Medical Research Council in its annual report for 1962–3.[1] This drew a distinction between research interventions intended to be of direct benefit to the subject of the research, and those that are not so intended. These two categories of research are generally called 'therapeutic' and 'non-therapeutic' research; there are difficulties and complications in such nomenclature which are discussed more fully in our next chapter. The MRC annual report stated that ' . . . in the strict view of the law parents and guardians of minors cannot give consent on their behalf to any procedures which are of no particular benefit to them and which may carry some risk of harm.' This statement was based on expert legal opinion and has regularly been interpreted as placing a complete embargo on non-therapeutic research on children. In 1982, a senior lecturer in paediatrics was for several months refused permission by the research ethics committee of his medical school for a research project that involved the taking of a single 2.5 ml blood sample from infants aged three to six months. Since the taking of the blood sample was not related to any treatment or diagnostic investigation needed by the infants, the lay member of the research ethics committee argued that, according to the Medical Research Council statement, such a procedure must be unlawful. Approval was eventually given by the committee after it had obtained another opinion of the presumed state of the law.

The first indication of a change in attitude away from a complete prohibition of research on children that was not intended directly to benefit them was given by the publication in 1973 of the report of the Royal College of Physicians 'Committee on the supervision of the ethics of clinical investigations in institutions'.[2] It stated: 'If advances in medical treatment are to continue so must clinical research investigation. It is in this light therefore that it is recommended that clinical research investigation of children or mentally handicapped adults which is not of direct benefit to the patient should be conducted, but only when the procedures entail negligible risk or discomfort and subject to the provisions of any common and statute law prevailing at the time. The parent or guardian should be consulted and his agreement recorded.' This appears to suggest that it is permissible to conduct non-therapeutic research on children, provided that it is perceived to be of negligible risk. There had, however, been no relevant change in the law since 1963, and the committee adduced no legal opinion to counter that of eminent counsel, upon which the earlier Medical Research Council statement had been based. When, indeed, the DHSS in 1975 issued its circular *Supervision of the ethics of clinical research investigations and fetal research,*[3] which included the Royal College of Physicians' recommendations, it drew attention to this point, warning Health Authorities '. . . that they ought not to infer from this recommendation that the fact that consent has been given by the parent or guardian and that the risk involved is considered negligible will be sufficient to bring such clinical research investigation within the law as it stands.' The then Chief Medical Officer also wrote elsewhere[14] that it was not legitimate to perform any experiment on a child that was not in the child's interests.

In 1975 therefore, the position with regard to therapeutic research on children remained much as it had been in 1865, when

Bernard wrote: 'It is our duty and our right to perform an experiment on man whenever it can save his life, cure him or gain him some personal benefit.'[11] The essential precaution that was necessary was stated in the 1975 revision of the Declaration of Helsinki: 'The potential benefits, hazards and discomfort of a new method should be weighed against the advantages of the best current diagnostic and therapeutic methods.' The Helsinki Declaration of 1975 is probably the most widely known and internationally accepted set of guidelines for the conduct of research on humans, having been prepared by the World Medical Association. Indeed, in the survey addressed to chairmen of research ethics committees undertaken by the working group, just over half found the Helsinki Declaration 'helpful' or 'very helpful', while only 2 per cent thought it unhelpful. Yet, in the matter of non-therapeutic research on children, or indeed on any other potential subjects deemed legally incompetent, it provides no clear guidance. In section III, 'Non-Therapeutic biomedical research involving human subjects' it states firmly that: 'The subjects should be volunteers', without suggesting that a parent or legal guardian might be able to volunteer a minor or legally incompetent person for such research. While there may be some older children who are competent to volunteer as subjects in research that is 'without direct diagnostic or therapeutic value' to them, this will not be true in general. It is not clear that the statement in section I, 'Basic principles', about the obtaining of consent to a proposed research procedure: '. . . when the subject is a minor, permission from the responsible relative replaces that of the subject . . .' was in any way intended to suggest that a responsible relative might also volunteer a child for non-therapeutic research. The final statement of the Declaration, concerning non-therapeutic research, 'In research on man, the interest of science and society should never take precedence over considerations related to the well-being of the subject' would seem to rule out the possibility of non-therapeutic research on a non-competent minor, unless all threat to the well-being of the subject were excluded. By definition, such research is not intended to be of benefit to the subject, and may therefore be, to a greater or less extent, detrimental to the well-being of the child. There is some evidence to suggest that children who volunteer for such research may coincidentally benefit by an increase in their self-esteem, but such a conclusion is not generalizable since such benefit is likely to be dependent on the degree of coercion – or lack of it – applied to any child subject.

At this point a paediatric researcher might well be left wondering what on earth he was to do when he wanted to proceed with some simple research project that unfortunately involved nontherapeutic research. Such a project might well be an attempt to establish the normal values of some biochemical variable, or the normal process of development, since, without a clear idea of normality, it becomes difficult both to recognize and to rectify abnormality. An example might be the establishment of a normal range for plasma amylase activity, which required a single blood sample from each of a group of normal children. Another example might be the physical examination of normal children, and careful questioning of their parents, about the natural history of micturition control and enuresis; it was the result of such surveys that led to a better understanding of the normal development of bladder control and a reduction in the number of children inappropriately treated for enuresis.

If the researcher consulted the Medical Research Council statement, he would have to conclude that he could not undertake either project. The Royal College of Physicians' report would permit him to go ahead with either project, until he read the DHSS circular, and realized that he might yet be acting unlawfully. The Helsinki Declaration would be unlikely to help him to make up his mind. It was in the midst of this confusion that the British Paediatric Association set up, in 1978, a working party on the ethics of research on children. The four members were all eminent academic paediatricians, and their report was published in 1980 as 'Guidelines to aid ethical committees considering research involving children'.[4] It marks a radical change in approach to the problems of non-therapeutic research on children, moving away from the apparently absolute prohibition of the MRC and the minor relaxation of such prohibition in the Royal College of Physicians' report to a permission that is qualified only to a relatively minor degree.

The British Paediatric Association guidelines are based on four premises, of which the first two are unexceptionable. They state:

> That research involving children is important for the benefit of all children and should be supported and encouraged, and conducted in an ethical manner.

That research should never be done on children if the same investigation could be done on adults.

The third premise is: 'That research which involves a child and is of no benefit to that child (non-therapeutic research) is not necessarily either unethical or illegal.' In view of the previous guidelines discussed above, and the lack of any change in statute or case law in the interim, this is a surprising statement, the more so since no evidence is presented to support the premise. Reference is made, without discussion, to a single paper[15] in which it was argued that courts were likely to take a more lenient view of the practice of non-therapeutic research on children than had hitherto been supposed.

The fourth premise states: 'That the degree of benefit resulting from a research should be assessed in relation to the risk of disturbance, discomfort or pain – the "Risk/Benefit ratio" ', and the rest of the guidelines are devoted mainly to an elaboration of this premise. They state explicitly, for instance, that more than negligible risk in non-therapeutic research on children may be justifiable provided that the anticipated benefits are sufficiently great, and their definition of 'negligible' allows what would widely be considered quite substantial risks to be classified as 'negligible'. Having divided risk into three categories, 'negligible', 'minimal', and 'more than minimal', and having asserted that no research ethics committee would countenance the risk of serious harm in any research procedure, the guidelines state: 'During the course of an abdominal operation, a renal biopsy might be taken for research purposes. The *Risk* here would be judged *More than Minimal* and the *Benefit* would have to be very large to justify it. But suppose the research aimed to resolve the problem of rejection of transplanted kidneys, with resulting lifesaving consequences both for children and adults with renal failure, this might be considered a *Benefit* of sufficient magnitude to justify the risk.' The guidelines give similar risk/benefit analyses to justify non-therapeutic blood sampling, including repeated glucose tolerance tests in diabetic children, where this might bring benefits to other diabetic children.

At first sight this may seem inconsistent with the earlier disclaimer that no ethical committee would accept a risk of possible serious harm to research subjects; after all, renal biopsies may occasionally result in appreciable morbidity or mortality. Admittedly, it is of low statistical probability, but the risk of a patient dying as a result of such investigations does exist. In this instance, however, the British Paediatric Association is not inconsistent, for it defines 'negligible risk' as 'risk less than that run in everyday life'. Many people would in fact regard the risks run in everyday life as substantial, both in terms of the lethal and disabling hazards faced, and in terms of the probabilities of those hazards occurring. (This distinction between degrees and probabilities of harmfulness is vital in risk assessment, but often blurred.) If everyday risks are to be regarded as the baseline for both, with 'risks less than that run in everyday life' being classified as 'negligible', 'risks questionably greater than negligible' being classified as 'minimal', and any greater risk being simply called 'more than minimal', then, of course, risk of significant morbidity and even mortality can properly be labelled 'negligible', for such risk is certainly a part of everyday life. It seems doubtful, however, that that was what was intended by the report of the Royal College of Physicians in 1973 when the RCP committee moved from the previous virtually absolute prohibition of non-therapeutic research on children to acceptance, provided that there was 'negligible risk or discomfort'. Regardless of the intention of the RCP report, however, one must ask whether such a degree of risk, and greater, can be a morally acceptable basis for non-therapeutic research on children. There is, indeed, a real inconsistency between the 1980 BPA guidelines and an editorial published in the Association's journal, *Archives of Disease in Childhood,* in 1978.[16] The editorial states that the only instance in which the journal has a definite policy not to accept papers is when ionizing radiations have been given to normal children for study purposes only. It continues: 'We could, of course, quote other investigations which would be regarded as obviously reasonable, e.g. weighing, or obviously unreasonable, if done for research purposes only, e.g. liver or renal biopsy. However, this is not particularly helpful because we imagine no one would expect us to decide otherwise in these situations.'

Another notable feature of the BPA guidelines is the absence – in contrast to all the other guidelines mentioned – of a specific assertion of the supremacy of the research subject's interests over the interests of others. This may be accidental, or it may be deliberate and consistent with a primary interest in 'the benefit of all children', and with a belief in the moral supremacy of risk/benefit analysis, in which case it marks an important change of approach. Such emphasis on a purely utilitarian risk/benefit analysis requires careful consideration, as will be shown in a later chapter on philosophical considerations.

The British Medical Association's *Handbook of medical ethics* for 1980[17] covers the subject of research on children in three short paragraphs that have remained unchanged in several subsequent editions and that add little to the advice of earlier guidelines. There is no attempt, for instance, to distinguish therapeutic from non-therapeutic research on children. Two statements are made, however, that many would consider to be highly contentious. Paragraph 4.6(b) states that 'Adequate background information must be provided to the local ethical committee to allow the scientific merit of the proposal to be judged as well as the ethics.' The extent of the role of research ethics committees in judging the scientific merit of proposals has been widely discussed. Many members of such committees would argue that, in general, the committees are not constituted in such a way as to have the necessary expertise to judge scientific merit. As will be discussed later, it is evident that to undertake a research project lacking in scientific merit is likely, for that reason, to be unethical, so that it should be a condition of ethical approval that any proposed research be judged scientifically valid. Such judgement, however, should be made by those competent to do so, which would frequently exclude the members of research ethics committees.

The same paragraph of the BMA's *Handbook of medical ethics* continues: 'The investigator should indicate the method he will use to obtain consent, i.e. from the parents and/or the general practitioner or consultant in charge of the case.' In other words, the BMA considers that there are occasions when an investigator may obtain consent from another doctor, whether general practitioner or consultant, for a research procedure to be carried out on a child, without any attempt to obtain either the child's or his parents' consent. Such a suggestion goes beyond even the BPA's relatively permissive guidelines in the licence it seeks to give doctors to carry out research on children. It seems highly unlikely, however, that a consent given by a doctor would carry any weight at all in the law courts, just as such a consent is largely devoid of any moral justification. Curiously enough, the notion that one might carry out research on children without attempting to obtain parental consent is taken a stage further in a recent British book *Law and medical ethics*[18] written by a doctor and a lawyer. Having suggested that it would be 'improper to proceed with an experiment involving a child against the wishes of its parents', they continue: 'The only exception might be when that refusal was clearly unreasonable and was jeopardising an otherwise essential trial; even then, a decision to go ahead should be taken only after very careful consideration.' Regardless of how essential a trial might be, or how carefully a researcher had considered his decision, following the above advice would be likely to have just one outcome for the researcher – an appearance in court on a charge of assault!

Before considering some of the guidelines for the conduct of research on children produced elsewhere, it is interesting to note the extent to which scientific experiments on animals are controlled in the United Kingdom. Whereas research on children has been controlled by voluntary adherence to guidelines only produced in the last twenty years or so, experiments on animals have had to comply with the requirements of the Cruelty to Animals Act since it became law in 1876. Both premises and researchers have had to be licensed by the Home Office, which has maintained a team of inspectors to ensure that the requirements of the Act are met. There has been regular discussion in various quarters of the adequacy of the current regulations, the most thorough such discussion being that of the Littlewood Committee.[19] One result has been the recent publication of a White Paper[20] which, if it becomes law, will further improve the protection of animals used in experiments.

In the United States of America, the National Commission for the Protection of Human Subjects of Biomedical and Behavioral Research was set up in 1974 with a mandate to develop ethical guidelines for the conduct of research on human subjects. In particular, it was required to examine various problems in research on children: its report and recommendations, *Research involving children*,[7] was published in 1977. In preparing its report, the Commission not only held many public hearings, but also commissioned substantial numbers of papers and reports, including a survey of the practice of over four hundred investigators engaged in research involving children between July 1974 and June 1975, and convened a national conference to ensure that the views of various minorities were heard. The report contains an analysis of the law as it applies to research on children and considerable discussion of the ethical bases of various viewpoints; it also includes some interesting arguments from members of the Commission who disagreed with some of the final recommendations.

The Commission's recommendations were generally fairly predictable. It found that research involving children was important for the health of all children, and that such research could be conducted ethically subject to general conditions such as are found in the Helsinki Declaration.[5] It recommended that research not involving greater than minimal risk might be conducted on children subject to suitable permission being obtained from parents and children, that research with greater than minimal risk might be conducted if it held out the prospect of direct benefit to the subjects, and that research not holding the prospect of benefit to the subjects might be conducted so long as the risk involved was no more than a minor increase over minimal. As will be seen later, these recommendations differ little from those produced by this working group. The one substantive difference lies in the Commission's sixth recommendation, which states that research not included in the above categories – i.e. research which carries no prospect of direct benefit to the subject, but carries a risk greater than a small increase over minimal – can be carried out provided that it has been approved by a national ethics advisory board and has been open to public review and comment. The remaining recommendations concern the obtaining of assent and consent, and provide protections for children who are wards of the state or else reside in institutions. These recommendations were finally, with some slight changes, adopted as federal regulations applicable from June 1983.[21]

The US National Commission appears to be the only organization outside the United Kingdom which has examined with any thoroughness the ethical problems of research on children. There are occasional reports such as that of Giertz,[22] who examined the way in which paediatric research is controlled in Sweden. The Australian College of Paediatrics produced a single-page report on the ethics of research in children[23] which was similar in approach to the British Paediatric Association guidelines.[4] The National Health and Medical Research Council of Australia has recently published a report of its working party on *Ethics in medical research*[24] which briefly considers research on children, but does so largely by a minor rewording of the Australian College of Paediatrics report. The Proposed International Guidelines for biomedical research involving human subjects[6] contain a brief but useful consideration of some aspects of research on children in its 'general survey' section. One statement, however, is almost as restrictive as the MRC Report for 1962–3, and suggests again the apparent difficulties in the concept of risk. In discussing both therapeutic and non-therapeutic research on children, it is stated that 'in the vast majority of situations, however, no intervention can be countenanced that involves any predictable risk to health or prospect of unreasonable psychological disturbance, physical discomfort or pain.' It will be shown later in this report (Chapter 5) that it is both possible and necessary to be much more precise in the way in which risk is discussed.

Moral dilemmas

A common feature of all the British guidelines discussed is that no attempt is made to provide ethical justification for the advice offered. One may trace through them a gradual change in the opinions given by academic lawyers of the legal status of research on children. The nearest attempt at a discussion of an ethical principle is provided by the BPA guidelines' discussion of risk/benefit analysis. Yet even that rests on a premise that would be unacceptable to many, and proceeds by developing an unusual hierarchy of risk set against a concept of benefit that is not quantified in any way.

One area of agreement between the various guidelines is that, in general, therapeutic research poses fewer problems than non-therapeutic research. Difficulties may yet arise, however, in the context of randomized controlled trials – when the subject receives a therapy chosen at random from the two or more that are being tested – and in innovative therapy – when a new therapy is tried out, but not as part of a formal research project. Randomized controlled trials are generally considered to be the most scientific way to compare possible treatments: for such a trial to be ethical, the researcher must be genuinely uncertain before the trial which of the treatments on trial is better. One problem that arises is the question whether it is ethical to ask for a subject's consent, or that of the subject's parent or guardian, when neither subject nor researcher knows which therapy is being consented to, since the subject will be assigned to a therapy at random. A further problem is that the perceptions of different doctors and researchers about the relative merits of therapies may differ substantially. An example of such a problem has arisen recently with the Medical Research Council trial of periconceptional vitamins for the prevention of neural tube defects in the fetus.[25,26] The difficulties that the organizers of the trial have faced are based on the perceptions that different groups have about previous trials in this field. The organizers have considered that there is no adequate scientific evidence that vitamins have any preventive effect, and they have therefore proposed a proper randomized controlled trial. Various groups of objectors, on the other hand, have said that while there may not be complete proof of the efficacy of vitamins, the evidence of efficacy is too strong for a randomized trial to be ethical, since some women at risk of having an infant with a neural tube defect would receive no vitamins.

Ideally, in clinical research, consent, risk, and benefit are vested in one individual. In research on legally competent adults, for instance, consent is obtained from, and risk borne and benefit, if any, gained by the same individual. In therapeutic research on children, risk and benefit are vested in the same child. In non-therapeutic research on children, however, the child bears the risk, while other children may gain the benefits, and a third party, with neither risk nor benefit, gives consent. Examples have already been given of the sort of project in which non-therapeutic research is attempting to define a normal range, whether of plasma amylase or the age at which children develop full bladder control. In other studies, the interventions may be much less innocuous, as for instance in an investigation of children born suffering from the consequences of intrauterine rubella infection. Some researchers in Finland wished to see whether the rubella virus persisted in the brains of these children, and so performed lumbar punctures on twenty-one such children.[27] Virus was found in none of the specimens of cerebrospinal fluid, while antibodies to the virus were found in the cerebrospinal fluid of one child, who then had a further two lumbar punctures. The report of this project was published in a British journal. The report contained no indication of approval by an ethics committee or of parental consent having been sought, though such safeguards may have been taken.

Such examples raise the problem of assessing risk/benefit ratios as noted earlier. But they raise other problems, too. Researchers often claim that it would be unethical not to do research that furthers our knowledge of children, and some go further, suggesting that there is a moral obligation on children to participate in research. On the other hand, it has been argued that any research on children violates their personal autonomy if they are incapable of giving informed consent. Thus, the question of consent, and of whether it should be provided by a child, his parents or some third party , becomes of crucial importance. Among the essentials of consent are that it should be freely given, and that the research subject should previously have been fully informed of the nature and possible consequences of the research. There is considerable doubt as to whether either of these essentials can be achieved when children are the subject of research. Indeed, the difficulties are illustrated by the way in which different authors have suggested ages varying from 5 to 16 years as being the age at which children are capable of behaving altruistically and giving consent. If, however, children are not considered capable of giving consent, then researchers must rely on the proxy consent of their parents or guardians, the validity of which has also been attacked.

The present study

The above review of current guidelines for research on children and of some of the moral dilemmas posed by it indicates that, while there have been several attempts to answer the question 'What is legal in research on children?' there has been no attempt in the United Kingdom to answer the question 'What is ethical in research on children?' For this reason the Society for the Study of Medical Ethics (now the Institute of Medical Ethics) decided to set up a working group to study the ethics of clinical research investigations on children. The Society, and its associated student Medical Groups, have pioneered the study, in the United Kingdom, of medical ethics using a multi-disciplinary approach. The moral problems of conducting research on children appeared to be a subject that needed thorough discussion which of necessity should be multi-disciplinary in character. The original purposes of the study were stated to be:

(a) to analyse the complex moral questions raised by clinical research involving children in particular;
(b) to review the moral basis of existing guidelines for the conduct of clinical research on children;
(c) to examine the workings of ethics committees when assessing paediatric research proposals;
(d) to identify broadly acceptable moral criteria, where these exist, for the conduct of such research;
(e) to produce a study document, containing ethical guidelines for the conduct of clinical research involving children, designed

    (i) for the guidance of members of research ethics committees and professional bodies involved in the preparation of guidelines,

    (ii) to be of assistance in the preparation of any future legislation,

    (iii) to enhance the quality of professional and public thinking on this subject.

In addition to the potential audience mentioned in the list of study purposes above, it is obviously hoped that this report may be of practical value to investigators carrying out research on children. Generous funding from the Leverhulme Trust had made possible this study, and the working group met at regular intervals over a period of three years starting in January 1982.

In the study purposes mentioned above, the possibility of future legislation is mentioned. There is a strong body, both of medical and legal opinion, that does not believe that additional legislation in this field could serve any useful purpose, but the possibility was raised by the House of Commons Social Services Committee, chaired by Mrs Renee Short, that recommended in 1980 'that the DHSS should arrange for further medico-legal discussion with a view to amending the law as it relates to research on newborn infants.'[28]

This study was not set up because the Society for the Study of Medical Ethics had any reason to believe that unethical or harmful research was being undertaken on children in the United Kingdom. It is interesting to note, however, that when the study was announced, various reporters from the medical and the lay press assumed that that was the reason for the study, and were most disappointed when the Society was unable to provide them with suitable horror stories. During the course of the study, many reports of research on children, undertaken in the United Kingdom and published in British journals, were examined and few were found that described a project that might have been unethical, though there were some projects that could be described as unkind. It was, however, disturbing to note the publication of several reports, in the same British journals, of research projects carried out overseas that would have been most unlikely to have received ethical approval from any British research ethics committee. Some examples are examined in greater detail in a subsequent chapter, but two may be mentioned here. A French researcher performed four lumbar punctures each on fifty-seven newborn babies in the first two weeks of life in an unsuccessful attempt to find biochemical support for a rather unlikely scientific theory about brain damage in infants.[29] An Indian team performed liver biopsies on twenty-nine children with biochemically normal liver function, because the children had siblings with Indian childhood cirrhosis, and the researchers were looking, unsuccessfully, for evidence to support the idea that that disease has some sort of genetic origin.[30] The one problem that has become apparent during the study is the frequency, in the United Kingdom, with which parents are not informed that their children are involved in a research project, and are not, therefore, asked for their consent to their children's involvement. This appears to happen most often when research on new-born infants is taking place. The working group was for instance sent an application for research ethics committee approval which stated, under the section 'How will informed consent be obtained and by whom?' that 'It has not been the policy in the Special Care Baby Unit at . . . for informed consent to be obtained for this type of study.'

Working group discussions

At an early stage of the working group's discussions, various decisions were taken as to the limits that the working group should impose on itself. The most important of these was that it should consider research on live-born children from the moment of birth up to the age of 16 years. Such a decision excluded research on the fetus, evidently a large and growing field of endeavour, that gives rise to a number of ethical problems. The working group recognizes that children exist as human beings both before and after these age limits, and also recognizes that, while there may be a continuous physiological spectrum between an unviable fetus and a viable infant, there is a legal difference, expressed in particular when the former may become an abortus.

It was suggested that the working group might confine its discussions to research that was physically invasive, but this was felt to place too great a restriction on discussion. Moreover, other sorts of research – even observational studies – could produce problems such as emotional or psychological sequelae in the children involved. It was also agreed that the risks generated in the course of practitioners acquiring skills, whether in a routine therapeutic setting or in research, were outside the remit of the working group, being an inevitable part of the practice of medicine.

It was apparent to the working group that no discussion of the ethics of research on children could be valuable unless it was firmly rooted in the current practice of such research. Throughout its discussions, therefore, the working group has tried to collect many examples of current research to illustrate points being discussed. These examples have come from the experience of members of the working group, from studies of the paediatric literature and from appeals to paediatric researchers placed in the medical journals. Similarly, although the group included four who were members of research ethics committees, it was felt that it would be useful to try to simulate the discussions of such a committee. For one of its regular meetings, therefore, the working group constituted itself as a research ethics committee, and examined five protocols for proposed paediatric research projects. Some of the ideas that arose during that meeting are included in the chapter on research ethics committees.

The subject that was discussed at greatest length, since it reappeared continually in discussions about a variety of topics, was the distinction between therapeutic and non-therapeutic research. The attempt to divide research into these two categories appears intuitively to be important in determining what research may ethically be undertaken, yet the attempt may always fail. The problem is discussed fully in the next chapter, in which definitions are given of various words and phrases used in this report.

The third chapter of the report examines the need for, and scope of, clinical research on children, since it is easy for researchers simply to assume a 'research imperative' – i.e. that any search for new knowledge is automatically worthwhile. An attempt is made to look at research on children in a wider perspective, socially and geographically. The following chapter examines two philosophical systems – utilitarianism and deontology – that underlie much discussion in medical ethics, and indicates how particular problems in research on children might be approached by moral philosophers. A frequent component of such ethical discussions is consideration of risk/benefit analysis. Risk/benefit analysis is a process in which considerable interest is now being shown in a variety of scientific fields, perhaps the most obvious example being in the assessment of the value of peaceful uses of nuclear energy. In medical research there has been little interest yet in precise application of risk/

benefit analysis, rather than intuitive assessments. In Chapter 5 of this report is gathered all the information that could readily be traced about the risks of research procedures, in order to encourage the development of more precise risk/benefit analysis of proposals for research on children. The sixth chapter discusses legal aspects of research on children, considering in particular the duties of parents to their children and the circumstances in which a valid consent may be given for research on children. One question that arises is whether children may themselves give a valid consent to research in which they are subjects. Chapter 7 considers evidence of the psychological development of children that is relevant to the determination of the ages at which they may be involved to varying degrees in decisions about proposed research procedures.

The working group felt that it was important to obtain evidence of the ways in which research ethics committees consider proposals for research on children. Since no information was available even to indicate what research ethics committees existed, an attempt was made first to locate all such committees in England and Wales. A survey was then undertaken by questionnaire that looked in general at the structures and methods of working of the committees, and in particular at their approaches to research projects involving child subjects: the results are reported in Chapter 8. The ninth chapter follows the progress of a research project from the first bright idea up to publication of the results, and tries to provide practical advice on how to avoid ethical pitfalls at the various stages. The final chapter summarizes the conclusions and recommendations of the working group.

References

1. Medical Research Council. Responsibility in investigations on human subjects. In *Report of the Medical Research Council for the year 1962–63*, pp.21–5. HMSO, London (1964).
2. Royal College of Physicians. *Supervision of the ethics of clinical research investigations in institutions.* Royal College of Physicians, London (1973).
3. Department of Health and Social Security. *Supervision of the ethics of clinical research investigations and fetal research.* HSC(IS)153. DHSS, London (1975).
4. British Paediatric Association. Guidelines to aid ethical committees considering research involving children. *Archs Dis. Childh.* **55,** 75–7 (1980).

5. World Medical Association. *Declaration of Helsinki.* Recommendations guiding physicians in biomedical research involving human subjects. (Adopted, Helsinki, 1964: amended, Tokyo, 1975 and Venice, 1983.)
6. Council for International Organizations of Medical Sciences. *Proposed international guidelines for biomedical research involving human subjects.* CIOMS, Geneva (1982).
7. National Commission for the Protection of Human Subjects of Biomedical and Behavioral Research. *Research involving children;* Report and recommendations: 77-0004; Appendix: 77-0005. DHEW, Washington DC (1977).
8. Beecher, H. K. Ethics and clinical research. *New Engl. J. Med.* **274,** 1354–60 (1966).
9. Pappworth, M. H. *Human guinea pigs.* Routledge & Kegan Paul, London (1967).
10. Hippocrates. The Oath. In *Hippocrates (vol I),* transl. W. H. S. Jones. Heinemann, London (1923).
11. Bernard, C. *An introduction to the study of experimental medicine (1865).* Translated by H. Greene, and reprinted in *Ethics in medicine* (eds. S. J. Reiser, A. J. Dyck, and W. J. Curran) pp.137–9. MIT Press, Cambridge, Mass. (1977).
12. German Reich. Circular of the Ministry of the Interior on directives concerning new medical treatments and scientific experiments on man (1931). Translated in *Int. Dig. Hlth Legisl. (Geneva)* **31,** 408–11 (1980).
13. The Nuremberg Code. Reprinted in *Dictionary of medical ethics* (2nd edn) (eds. A. S. Duncan, G. R. Dunstan, and R. B. Welbourn) pp.130–2. Darton, Longman, & Todd, London (1981).
14. Godber, G. Constraints upon the application of medical advances. *Proc. R. Soc. Med.* **67,** 1273–312, at p.1311 (1974).
15. Dworkin, G. Legality of consent to non-therapeutic medical research on infants and young children. *Archs Dis. Childh.* **53,** 443–6 (1978).
16. Editorial. Research involving children – ethics, the law and the climate of opinion. *Archs Dis. Childh.* **53,** 441–2 (1978).
17. British Medical Association. *The handbook of medical ethics,* pp.25–6. BMA, London (1980).
18. Mason, J. K., and McCall Smith, R. A. *Law and medical ethics,* p.211. Butterworths, London (1983).
19. Departmental Committee on Experiments in Animals: *Report.* Cmnd 2641, HMSO, London (1965).
20. *Scientific procedures on living animals.* Cmnd 8883, HMSO, London (1983).
21. Department of Health and Human Services. 45CFR Part 46 Additional protections for children involved as subjects in research. *Federal Register (Washington DC)* **48,** 9814–20 (1983).
22. Giertz, G. Ethical aspects of paediatric research. *Acta paediat. scand.* **72,** 641–50 (1983).

23. Australian College of Paediatrics. Report on the ethics of research in children. *Aust. Paediat. J.* **17**, 162 (1981).
24. National Health and Medical Research Council. *Ethics in medical research*. Australian Government Publishing Service, Canberra (1983).
25. Editorial. Vitamins, neural-tube defects, and ethics committees. *Lancet* **i**, 1061–2 (1980).
26. Wynn, J. Spina bifida: Trials ahead. *Nature, Lond.* **299**, 198 (1982).
27. Vesikari, T., Meurman, O. H., and Maki, R. Persistent rubella-specific IgM-antibody in the cerebrospinal fluid of a child with congenital rubella. *Archs Dis. Childh.* **55**, 46–8 (1980).
28. Social Services Committee, Second Report. *Perinatal and neonatal mortality,* Vol. I. HMSO, London (1980).
29. Dalens, B., Viallard, J-L, Raynaud, E-J, Dastugue, B. CSF levels of lactate and hydroxybutyrate dehydrogenase as indicators of neurological sequelae after neonatal brain damage. *Devl Med. & Child Neurol.* **23**, 228–33 (1981).
30. Nayak, N. C., Marwaha, N., Kalra, V., Roy, S., and Ghai, O. P. The liver in siblings of patients with Indian childhood cirrhosis: a light and electron microscopic study. *Gut* **22**, 295–300 (1981).

2

Definitions

Research

Scientific language contains many words for which extremely precise single meanings are agreed; most of the technical words used in medicine are equally precise. The meanings of words used by moral philosophers are often less immediately certain, and indeed whole schools of philosophical thought have been built around attempts to find precise definitions of a few key words. The language of medical ethics lies inevitably between these extremes; curiously, however, some of the words most difficult to define are those which appear at first sight just to be technical terms. On several occasions members of our working group found that the meanings that they had always given to particular words were not accepted by other members. The most important example of this, in terms of the working group's discussions, was its lack of a common understanding of the meanings of 'therapeutic research' and 'non-therapeutic research', which will be discussed later in this chapter. First, however, some other words frequently used are considered.

Research may be defined as in the *Shorter Oxford English Dictionary:* 'An investigation directed to the discovery of some fact by careful study of a subject; a course of critical or scientific inquiry.' The second part of that definition is more useful when considering medical research, because of the potential confusion, caused by the use of the word 'investigation' in the first part. 'Investigation' tends to be used more specifically in medical practice to denote the ascertainment of a particular anatomical, biochemical, or physiological value in a patient. Examples of such 'investigations' are a chest X-ray, the measurement of the haemoglobin level in blood, or lung function tests. In our discussions, however, 'research' was seldom used by itself, without some other word attached. Phrases such as 'research project', 'research procedure', or 'therapeutic research' were used more frequently.

A *research project* is a systematic enquiry designed to contribute to generalizable knowledge. It is important to emphasize that it is systematic in design and execution, and requires honest and accurate recording of all information obtained. A speculative or haphazard attempt at a new therapy, for instance, cannot be regarded as a research project.

A *research intervention* is a specific act performed on a research subject during the course of a research project. Such an intervention may involve the performance of an investigation, used in the medical sense noted above, such as the taking of a blood sample or the measurement of lung function tests, or even simply weighing the subject. Alternatively, an intervention might be manipulation of the subject's diet, or the giving of a substance.

Research interventions may be either *invasive* or *non-invasive*. Essentially, any activity, part or all of which involves an entrance of any sort into a subject's body, is invasive. For instance, urine may be collected by both invasive and non-invasive techniques. If a urine bag is attached to an infant to collect urine voided normally, that is a non-invasive intervention, even though it may cause the infant some discomfort. If on the other hand the urine is collected by supra-pubic aspiration – that is, by passing a needle through the abdominal wall into the bladder and withdrawing some urine – the intervention is invasive. The borderline between invasive and non-invasive may sometimes be difficult to ascertain. Swabbing the skin so as to obtain a sample of bacteria growing thereon is a non-invasive intervention; swabbing the throat for similar purposes, while not involving the breaking of any skin or tegument, should be regarded as an invasive intervention.

Some research projects do not involve any interventions and consist only in *observation*. The *Concise Oxford English Dictionary* defines an observation as 'accurate watching and noting of phenomena as they occur in nature with regard to cause and effect or mutual relations', and it is in that sense that 'observation' has been used in this report. In medical research such 'accurate watching' might just be of the colour of a subject's skin, or the size of the pupils of his eyes. Were the pulse to be measured by feeling it at the wrist, that would constitute an intervention rather than an observation. Pure observation is an activity more commonly found in psychological research, particularly that undertaken by human ethologists, when the behaviour of one or more subjects is observed and recorded.

A *research procedure* is any act undertaken as part of a research project, and may consist in either an observation or an intervention, or a combination of the two.

The *Shorter Oxford English Dictionary* defines *therapy* as 'the medical treatment of disease; curative medical treatment'. While such a definition is admirably succinct, it may be too narrow, particularly when the derived adjective 'therapeutic' is used in the context of research. It is helpful to consider as therapy all the elements of a doctor's duty of care to his patient. In particular, this duty must include the process needed to arrive at a diagnosis before initiating treatment. Thus, all the elements of the normal medical process – history-taking, examination, observation, investigations, making a diagnosis, and assessing the prognosis – may be parts of therapy, although not necessarily 'curative medical treatment' in themselves. There would be dangers, however, in using quite such a broad definition as the Helsinki Declaration,[1] which includes '. . . saving life, re-establishing health or alleviating suffering'. The dangers would lie in the use of the word 'health', which the World Health Organisation regards as complete physical, mental, and social well-being. Such an all-embracing concept of health could allow a variety of activities to be classified as therapy, because to a greater or less extent, they 're-established health'. Even the taking of a blood sample for no reason related to a child's condition could be called therapy, since it might encourage the child to accept his social obligation to help others. In this report, 'therapy' is understood to include diagnosis, but not such a broad concept as that suggested above.

Therapeutic versus non-therapeutic

The terms '*therapeutic research*' and '*non-therapeutic research*' are commonly used to represent a perceived distinction between research that may benefit its subject (therapeutic), and research undertaken only to gain scientific knowledge (non-therapeutic). The distinction may often be of considerable practical value, being used both by commentators on the ethics of research on children, and in the formulation of guidelines and codes of ethics. All too often, however, such commentators and even some formulators of guidelines fail to define the terms before using them: while it is relatively easy to come to an intuitive understanding of the distinction, it is in practice extremely difficult to define the terms precisely and to apply them with certainty to every research project. One relatively simple expression of the distinction suggests that in therapeutic research the subject accepts the risks of research for his own benefit, while in non-therapeutic research he does so for the benefit of others. Other attempts to distinguish therapeutic research and non-therapeutic research rely on an assessment of the intention(s) of the researcher in a particular project.

There are those who would argue that the maintenance of a distinction between therapeutic research and non-therapeutic research serves no purpose. It is therefore intended to examine the way in which this distinction has developed, some of the attempts at definitions that have been produced by various bodies including this working group, and some of the difficulties encountered in applying the distinction to actual research projects.

That there have been for a very long time experiments on man that fall into the categories of therapeutic or non-therapeutic research is well known. Hippocrates[2] provides probably the earliest description of non-therapeutic research when describing a man with a fractured skull. As spicules of bone were removed, the underlying brain was stroked, and the convulsive movements of the opposite side of the body observed. It was noted above, in the introductory chapter, that Claude Bernard[3] distinguished between experiments that might be of benefit to the subject, and those that might be harmful to him, only the former being permissible. Similarly in 1931, German guidelines[4] distinguished therapeutic and non-therapeutic research, although they used the expressions innovative therapy and scientific experiment to describe the two categories.

Until the Second World War, the distinction between therapeutic and non-therapeutic research, while recognized, did not play a major part in discussions of what research was permissible. It was in the aftermath of the Nuremberg Military Tribunals, and the writing of the 'Nuremberg Code', that it started to assume a major importance. There was, rightly, a sense of outrage at the sorts of experiments conducted by doctors and scientists under orders from the Nazis on inmates of concentration camps and on other prisoners. Some of these were described by

Ivy[5] who had been asked by the US Government to investigate the experimental records. In particular he said, 'One of the experiments they performed, which was particularly atrocious, was the typhus experiment.' Prisoners in Buchenwald concentration camp were first injected with various experimental vaccines against typhus, and then, several weeks later, with blood from a patient with typhus. Within days three-quarters of the prisoners were dead, the only exception being one group who had received the 'Weigl' vaccine, of whom half had died.

One result of revelations such as this was the drawing up of the Nuremberg Code.[6] This laid great emphasis on the need to protect the rights of every individual research subject, regardless of the potential value to society of a research project. It started by emphasizing that 'the voluntary consent of the human subject is absolutely essential' and continued by noting the need for a rigorous assessment of possible risks and benefits in any research project. A further result, however, was the development, both in the research community and amongst commentators, of an attitude which called into question all research that was not designed to be of benefit to the subject. This was particularly true when research on children was considered, and found expression, for instance, in the Medical Research Council's report for 1962–3[7] quoted in the introductory chapter, and in the writings of Paul Ramsey,[8,9] an eminent American moral theologian. Unfortunately, the opposite attitude has also become apparent: that any research, on children or adults, is acceptable, so long as one can call it therapeutic research. An extreme example of this attitude is illustrated by a project reported to the Association of European Paediatric Cardiologists in May 1983.[10] A group of paediatric cardiologists in Paris tried out a new procedure for correction of a congenital anatomical defect of the vessels of the heart, called transposition of the great arteries; it is a defect for which two standard procedures, the Senning and the Mustard, are already available, with mortality ranging from zero to 10 per cent in large paediatric cardiology centres. The new Parisian procedure was carried out in two stages: six out of thirty children (20 per cent) died in the first stage, and two more were saved by having the standard Senning procedure undertaken as an emergency. In the second stage a further seven children died, giving an overall mortality of 43 per cent; nine children were finally asymptomatic, but of these five were thought still to have abnormal cardiac function. The response of the researchers to such high mortality and morbidity was not to abandon their two-stage procedure, but to decide to try it out on much younger infants, preferably within one week of birth.

A further problem raised by the distinction between therapeutic and non-therapeutic research is that application of the distinction may lead to two different standards of consent. This problem in particular led the Canadian Medical Research Council, in its 'Report of the working group on human experimentation',[11] to drop the distinction as explained in the following extract:

> 'Although this distinction is often relevant in evaluating risk and benefit, it is important to recognize that such a division can create harmful misconceptions. This dichotomy implies that therapeutic research will have some direct benefit on the patient . . . As a result the need for full and careful consent, considered to be so important in non-therapeutic research, is often glossed over because therapeutic research is confounded with treatment or care.'

The well-known experiments at the Willowbrook State School in New York[12,13] provide a further example of the difficulties that can arise, when trying to use the distinction. The school was an institution whose inmates were 5000 mentally retarded children; various infections, including viral hepatitis and measles, were endemic. Studies were undertaken to increase knowledge of the natural history of hepatitis and to try to produce immunity to it. New entrants to the school, who had not previously suffered from hepatitis, were admitted to a special unit segregated from the rest of the school. There they were either injected with, or given oral doses of, virus-containing extracts of faeces from children who already had viral hepatitis, so as to induce the disease.

Obviously, such a project raises many ethical problems, not least because the International Code of Medical Ethics[14] states that 'Any act or advice which could weaken physical or mental resistance of a human being may be used only in his interest.' It is also interesting to compare this experiment with the Nazi typhus experiment described earlier. Moreover, it would appear that this project must consist in non-therapeutic research, since one is actually giving a child an illness. The researchers argued, however, during the considerable controversy that not surprisingly arose after publication of several papers, that their research was of benefit to the subjects. The latter were in a segregated unit in which they were not exposed to measles, shigellosis, and various parasitic and respiratory infections endemic in the school. Had they not been isolated, they would have been exposed to the virus in the school; giving the virus in a controlled way meant that 'they were likely to have a subclinical infection followed by immunity to the particular hepatitis virus'.[15] Thus, there is considerable difficulty in knowing whether to assign the project to the category of non-therapeutic, or of therapeutic, research. Some members of the working group found this series of experiments extremely objectionable, and felt that the experiments must therefore be classified as non-therapeutic. It is important to note, however, that one cannot judge whether research is therapeutic or not just by deciding how objectionable one thinks it to be.

The working group spent a long time discussing the possible distinction between therapeutic and non-therapeutic research, its value in practice, and ways in which it might be defined. The example given illustrates some of the difficulties in making the distinction in practice. These difficulties were faced also by the US National Commission for the Protection of Human Subjects of Biomedical and Behavioral Research. While they found it easy to accept the value of research conducted in the context of therapy, they felt that a total acceptance of such 'therapeutic research' would allow too much research of questionable ethical propriety. They therefore decided to define more precisely their categories of research, and arrived at:

(a) 'research . . . by an intervention that holds out the prospect of direct benefit for the individual subjects, or by a monitoring procedure required for the well-being of the subjects', and

(b) 'research . . . by an intervention that does not hold out the prospect of direct benefit for the individual subjects, or by a monitoring procedure not required for the well-being of the subjects.'[16]

One has to agree with McCartney[17] that it would have been simpler had the Commission defined the former as therapeutic research and the latter as non-therapeutic research rather than using such unwieldy phrases throughout their recommendations. It is interesting to note however that the expressions 'therapeutic research' and 'non-therapeutic research' nevertheless appear frequently in the report and its appendix, indicating their essential usefulness. The problem remains that the maintenance of the distinction between therapeutic and non-therapeutic research promotes the idea that research designed to make people better is intrinsically less problematical than research designed to improve basic knowledge. In reality, it may often be the case, though obviously open to argument, that fundamental scientific and medical research is of more value in the long term than therapeutic research; and that children are sometimes less protected in therapeutic research than in non-therapeutic research.

Controls

A further problem that arises in employing the distinction is that of allocating the 'controls' used in a project either to therapeutic or to non-therapeutic research. Controls are subjects who are used for the purposes of comparison. In a trial of a new drug, for instance, the subjects may be chosen at random to receive either the drug or an inert substance, a placebo. Those receiving the placebo act as controls, since they will come under all the same influences – whether pathological, environmental or psychological – as the subjects, except for the influence of the drug that is on trial. Provided that neither the subject nor the researcher knows whether the drug or the placebo is being taken, an objective assessment may be made of any effects that are specifically attributable to the drug. Such a trial is called a double-blind randomized controlled trial and examples will be discussed later in the report.

Another sort of control may be a normal child, some aspect of whose anatomy, biochemistry, physiology, or psychology is to be compared with that of a child suffering from a particular illness. An example of the use of this sort of control is provided by a recent paper with the splendidly ambiguous title 'Anorectal manometry results in defecation disorders'.[18] The purpose of the reported project was to try to establish whether anorectal manometry – the measurement of pressures at various levels of the anus and rectum – and rectal biopsy '. . . have a useful role in the diagnosis, prediction of response to conservative management, and prognosis of children with constipation or faecal soiling.' Forty-seven children with these defecation disorders, and eleven control children, 'none of whom had a history of bowel dysfunction or neurological disorder', were investigated. A metal probe was passed so that rubber-covered chambers, formed in the probe at 1 cm intervals, lay in the anal canal; a rubber balloon nearer the tip of the probe lay in the rectum. The balloon was then blown up and the changes in pressure in the anal canal recorded from the rubber covered chambers. After this had been done two or three times, suction biopsies were taken from three different parts of the rectum. The ages of the controls ranged from seven months to sixteen years; 'small children occasionally required sedation or ketamine anaesthesia'. The project was approved by the district research ethics committee, but the paper does not mention whether informed consent was obtained from the parents. For the present, it is enough to note that child controls can have quite invasive procedures performed on them, and may even be anaesthetized in order that such procedures may be performed; the other questions raised by this project will be discussed later in the report. Since the child controls in this example had no relevant bowel or neurological disorder, the procedures could not be intended to benefit them, and it is therefore clear that they were involved in non-therapeutic research, even though the subject children were participating in therapeutic research. On the other hand, it is sometimes argued that one should only consider a project as a whole, so that this project would be a therapeutic research project since it held out the prospect of benefit at least to some of the children involved.

A further sort of control is that employed in a comparison of drug regimes. In the treatment of acute lymphoblastic leukaemia, for instance, the control children may receive what is considered to be the best treatment regime – generally a mixture of three or four cytotoxic drugs, possibly with the addition of selective radio-therapy – while the subject children receive a new regime which might be an improvement. Now that the cure rate for acute lymphoblastic leukaemia (ALL) is greater than 50 per cent, one may quite reasonably claim that both groups are receiving therapeutic benefit and that such a trial constitutes therapeutic research. Twenty years ago, however, one might have come to a different conclusion, the two-year survival rate then for children with ALL being less than 10 per cent. Children entered into a trial of treatment regimes with that sort of prognosis were almost certain to be dead before the trial had ended, so that future cohorts of children with ALL might benefit, but those in the trial were most unlikely to. It is therefore relevant to ask whether such a trial was therapeutic or non-therapeutic research; and the question remains relevant since other malignant tumours, for which treatment regimes are being tried, still have such poor prognoses – stage III or IV neuro-blastoma, hepatoblastoma, or rhabdomyosarcoma, for instance.[19]

The working group's definitions

In spite of the various practical difficulties in the use of a distinction between therapeutic and non-therapeutic research, the working group decided to persevere in its attempt to formulate a definition of the distinction that would take into account as many as possible of the difficulties. It did so because there are certain practical advantages in retaining the distinction. For instance, although considerations of risk and benefit can play no part in the definition, the distinction itself may play an important role in weighing the risks against the benefits of a particular project. The distinction is also of relevance when deciding on the need for consent: while it is certain that informed consent, either of a subject or else of the parent or guardian of a child subject, is needed before the performance of a non-therapeutic research procedure, there may be occasions, particularly in emergencies, when the need for informed consent to therapeutic research may be waived. The concept of doing research during an emergency may at first seem rather odd, but there are occasions, such as the case mentioned at the start of this report, when it will be necessary to compare a proposed new treatment for the emergency against the existing treatment.

The working group examined *inter alia* previous definitions produced by the United States National Institutes of Health,[20] a Ciba Foundation study group,[21] and the World Medical Association in the Helsinki Declaration.[1] While each came close to expressing what the working group felt to be the essential distinction between therapeutic and non-therapeutic research none defined carefully enough the intention of the researcher. The central point is that since therapy is distinguished from research by the intention of the person doing it, research can never be, in itself, therapy.

Therefore the distinction has to be that *therapeutic research* is research consisting in an activity which has also a therapeutic intention, as well as a research intention, towards the subjects of the research, and *non-therapeutic research* is research activity which has not also a therapeutic intention.

A therapeutic intention is to have as one's purpose therapy, in the sense discussed earlier in this chapter.

This definition of the distinction between therapeutic and non-therapeutic research was approved by the working group because it makes clear the dual intent of therapeutic research. It was also argued, however, that such dual intent was unlikely or even impossible; a researcher would always have the primary intent of gaining new knowledge. Such a suggestion seems improbable, however: in reality, a researcher would be using his clinical and therapeutic acumen in the interests of the research element of his activity, at the same time as using his research skills for the clinical benefit of his research subject. If one invites friends round for dinner, one has the dual intent of feeding them and talking with them: it would indeed be a strange occasion if one fed them only without saying a word the whole evening; or vice versa!

One research proposal examined by the working group illustrates both the need in some circumstances to decide whether a project is therapeutic or non-therapeutic, and the difficulties that may be met in so deciding. The proposal had been submitted to the working group by the chairman of a research ethics committee which had been in difficulty when trying to decide whether or not to approve the proposal.

The purpose of the project was to study water fluxes in sick pre-term infants and to assess in particular the insensible water gain from humidifiers attached to artificial ventilators, and the insensible water loss from the lungs and skin. Ten infants requiring artificial ventilation for hyaline membrane disease would be studied. In such infants, water balance is very important in determining the development of several potentially fatal complications, but little is known about insensible water gain or loss from the respiratory tract in particular. In the study, deuterium oxide, heavy water or D_2O, would be added to the humidifier water in the artificial ventilator. Its accumulation in the neonate could then be followed by measuring the proportion of D_2O to ordinary water, H_2O, in blood samples taken sequentially. These blood samples would be very small, since only five microlitres (about one-twentieth of a drop) of blood would be required in order to measure D_2O by mass spectrometry; they would be taken – over a period of three days, and with no discomfort – from an umbilical arterial catheter, which is usually inserted when infants are artificially ventilated.

The problem that had arisen with this proposal concerned the obtaining of parental consent. The policy in the special care baby unit where the proposed project would be undertaken was not to obtain informed consent for this type of study. The researchers therefore proposed to dispense with informed consent, while the research ethics committee thought that it should be obtained.

One reason why it is necessary to establish whether such a project is therapeutic or non-therapeutic is a legal one. The removal of blood samples from the infants would be an assault unless consent had been given. Although there is no specific statement of the law in such circumstances, it is likely that the courts would always regard unconsented invasive non-therapeutic research as unlawful. They might take a somewhat more lenient view of unconsented therapeutic research, though not necessarily.

The basic difficulty in considering whether or not this project is therapeutic research is to decide whether there is a therapeutic intention towards the infant subjects. It is essential to provide humidified air to infants on artificial ventilators: one argument therefore states that the addition of D_2O to humidifier water merely alters slightly one therapeutic activity without in any way altering the therapeutic intention. It is a necessary part of medical practice to examine the results of therapies that are used in order that they may be improved: such assessment of a therapy is inevitably therapeutic research.

Another view would suggest that the addition of D_2O to humidifier water is not a necessary part of therapy, and is not intended, in itself, to be therapy. The taking of additional blood samples – even though they amount to a very small total quantity – is not a therapeutic activity; the researchers have not stated how soon the measurements of D_2O might be made, and nowhere in their protocol have they suggested that the measurements might be used to improve the control of water balance in the infant subjects. The project is therefore designed to gain physiological knowledge, and there is no therapeutic intention towards the infant subjects in the proposed activities that are additional to standard therapy.

The problem of deciding which argument is correct seems finally to be insoluble. In terms of the definitions adopted by the working group (referred to on p. 33) it is possible, however, to conclude that this is a therapeutic research project since the researchers have both a therapeutic intention, in humidifying the air supplied by the ventilators, and a research intention. It is not suggested that the definitions adopted by the working group will solve all the problems with which research ethics committees are in practice faced.

The researchers in the anorectal manometry project,[18] for instance, had no therapeutic intention towards the controls that they used. To identify the controls as taking part in therapeutic research because there was a therapeutic intention towards the subjects of the research project seems invidious and inherently inequitable. In some circumstances it may then be important to abandon attempts to describe a whole research project as either therapeutic or non-therapeutic, and to consider instead the nature of the actual procedures undertaken. In this case, the subjects had therapeutic interventions performed on them, while the controls had non-therapeutic interventions performed.

The definitions adopted by the working group allow firm conclusions to be reached about some other projects mentioned earlier. When the Willowbrook experiments started, there was no therapeutic intention in them towards the handicapped subjects, although some benefits may have accrued to them incidentally. By the working group's definitions, they were therefore non-therapeutic research projects. On the other hand, the comparative trials of treatment regimes for leukaemia and other malignancies were and are therapeutic research, since there has always been a therapeutic intention towards each of the subjects, even when the major benefits would probably fall to later cohorts. The definitions also obviate the need for such complicating expressions as 'partly therapeutic', that have been suggested to describe an intervention such as the taking of an additional two millilitres of blood for a research purpose, when a blood specimen is to be taken anyway as part of therapy. Since the act of taking the blood sample has both a therapeutic and a research intention, the act is therapeutic – by definition.

Innovative therapy

One final class of activity needs to be considered in a chapter of definitions: innovative therapy. *Innovative therapy* consists in the performance of a new or non-standard intervention as all or part of a therapeutic activity and not as part of a formal research project. Innovative therapy may therefore be quite haphazard, starting just when a doctor has a bright idea that he wants to try out. If the bright idea seems to be any good, then innovative therapy can become research as soon the bright idea is examined in a systematic manner. Much innovative therapy is surgical in nature, since surgeons often try out modifications to existing surgical procedures and occasionally try out new operations. It is rare for these modifications or new operations to be undertaken as part of a formal research project and they have not in general been subject first to peer review or review by a research ethics committee. Another sort of innovative therapy would be the introduction of new instruments, if these were not formally compared with existing ones. Innovative therapy is comparatively rare in the use of medicines, but it can still occur. A doctor may decide that a drug that is already available for the treatment of one disease might be useful in the treatment of another, and he is at liberty within the limits of his professional expertise to go ahead and try it. One example a few years ago was the use of injectable phenothiazine drugs. These were introduced to help in the treatment of schizophrenia, their value being that a schizophrenic could have his illness controlled by a monthly injection. Doctors looking after mentally handicapped children with severe behaviour disturbances realized that these drugs might help: it was found that monthly injections of quite small doses produced considerable improvement in the behaviour of the few children in whom the drugs were tried. It was then decided to set up a controlled trial to discover whether the results were real: i.e. what started as innovative therapy became therapeutic research as the trial was set up, and the haphazard procedures became formalized.

A more recent example of innovative therapy is the description of the treatment of four patients, three of them children, with potentially fatal meningococcal septicaemia.[22] During an epidemic of meningococcal disease in northern Norway, half of the patients admitted to one hospital who developed fulminant septicaemia died despite intensive conventional treatment. Since many of the life-threatening effects of this bacterium are caused by a toxic substance, an endotoxin, produced by the bacterium, it was decided to try to remove the endotoxin from the blood stream of affected patients. This was done in the three older patients by plasmapheresis and leucapheresis, a process by which the red cells in the patient's blood are separated from the rest of the blood (the plasma and the leucocytes) and then returned to the patient mixed with fresh frozen plasma from a donor. In the youngest child, an exchange transfusion was undertaken, i.e. 20 ml of the patient's blood was removed, and replaced with the same volume of fresh blood, this process being repeated many times. All four patients recovered without any after-effects, although previous experience during the epidemic suggested that three of the patients would have died if given conventional treatment only. The new treatment therefore seems likely to be very useful, but the authors state in their conclusions that the 'future place of this treatment, however, must be determined by clinical trials'.

References

1. World Medical Association. *Declaration of Helsinki.* Recommendations guiding physicians in biomedical research involving human subjects. (Adopted, Helsinki, 1964; amended, Tokyo, 1975 and Venice, 1983.)
2. Hippocrates. On wounds in the head. In *Hippocrates (vol III),* transl. E. T. Withington. Heinemann, London (1927).
3. Bernard, C. *An introduction to the study of experimental medicine (1865).* Transl. H. Greene, and reprinted in *Ethics in medicine* (eds. S. J. Reiser, A. J. Dyck, and W. J. Curran) pp.257-9. MIT Press, Cambridge, Mass. (1977).
4. German Reich. Circular of the Ministry of the Interior on directives concerning new medical treatments and scientific experiments on man (1931). Translated in *Int. Dig. Hlth Legisl. (Geneva)* **31,** 408-11 (1980).
5. Ivy, A. C. Nazi war crimes of a medical nature. *Fed. Bull.* **33,** 133-46 (1947).
6. The Nuremberg Code. Reprinted in *Dictionary of medical ethics* (2nd edn) (eds. A. S. Duncan, G. R. Dunstan, and R. B. Welbourn) pp.130-2. Darton, Longman, & Todd, London (1981).
7. Medical Research Council. Responsibility in investigations on human subjects. In *Report of the Medical Research Council for the year 1962-63,* pp.21-5. HMSO, London (1964).
8. Ramsey, P. *The patient as person,* pp.1-58. Yale University Press, New Haven and London (1970).
9. ——. The enforcement of morals: non-therapeutic research on children. *Hastings Center Report* **6**(4), 21-30 (1976).
10. Sidi, D., Cachaner, J., Hazan, E., Lecompte, Y., Fermont, L., and Villain, E. Anatomical correction of simple transposition of the great arteries; results of two-stage procedure in 30 cases. *Paediat. Cardiol.* (In press.).
11. Medical Research Council (Canada). *Ethical considerations in research involving human subjects.* MRC, Ottawa (1978).
12. Ward, R., Krugman, S., Giles, J. P., Jacobs, A. M., and Bodansky, O. Infectious hepatitis: studies of its natural history and prevention. *New Engl. J. Med.* **258,** 407-16 (1958).
13. Krugman, S., Ward, R., Giles, J. P., Bodansky, O., and Jacobs, A. M. Infectious hepatitis: detection of the virus during the incubation period and in clinically inapparent infection. *New Engl. J. Med.* **261,** 729-34 (1959).

14. World Medical Association. *International code of medical ethics* (1949). Reprinted in *The handbook of medical ethics*, pp.57–9. British Medical Association, London (1980).
15. Krugman, S. Experiments at the Willowbrook State School (letter). *Lancet* **i**, 966–7 (1971).
16. National Commission for the Protection of Human Subjects of Biomedical and Behavioral Research. *Research involving children*, Report and recommendations: 77-0004. DHEW, Washington DC (1977).
17. McCartney, J. J. Research on children: National commission says 'Yes, if . . .' *Hastings Center Report* **8**(5), 26–31 (1978).
18. Molnar, D., Taitz, L. S., Urwin, O. M., and Wales, J. K. H. Anorectal manometry results in defecation disorders. *Archs Dis. Childh.* **58**, 257–61 (1983).
19. Morris-Jones, P. Current approaches to cancer in childhood. In *Recent advances in paediatrics*, vol. 6 (ed. D. Hull) pp.179–94. Churchill Livingstone, Edinburgh (1981).
20. Department of Health, Education and Welfare: National Institutes of Health. Protection of human subjects, policies and procedures. *Federal Register (Washington DC)* **38**, 31738–49 (1973).
21. Ciba Foundation Study Group. Medical research: civil liability and compensation for personal injury – a discussion paper. *Br. med. J.* **i**, 1172–5 (1980).
22. Bjorvatn, B., Bjertnaes, L., Fadnes, H. O., Flaegstad, T., Gutteberg, T. J., Kristiansen, B-E, Pape, J., Rekvig, O. P., Osterud, B., and Aanderud, L. Meningococcal septicaemia treated with combined plasmapheresis and leucapheresis or with blood exchange. *Br. med. J.* **288**, 439–41 (1984).

3

Child health and the scope of research

Why child health has improved

In the early 1850s, A.C. Tait, who later became a much-respected Archbishop of Canterbury, was Dean of Carlisle. While in Carlisle, his wife developed scarlet fever and died of it. In those days it was the custom always for close relatives to kiss the departed immediately after death. Over the next few weeks each of the Dean's five daughters in turn developed scarlet fever and died of it. Only he and his son survived.

That such a story would now be impossible in the developed world is but one indication of the great improvements in health and medical care that have occurred in little over a century. It is important to realize that such improvements are the result of many different factors, social and economic as well as medical. It is unlikely, for instance, that a modern family would be so large – few Deans have six children today – so fewer people would be at risk of contracting the infection. General levels of health and nutrition are better nowadays, so that each individual's ability to resist the disease is greater and the disease is less likely to be fatal, even if untreated. In medical terms, the great advances have been in the recognition of bacteria as the cause of infections like scarlet fever, and the development of antibiotics for their treatment. Thus, penicillin is available to treat the streptococcal infection that is the basis of scarlet fever, so that the illness is seldom more severe nowadays than a sore throat with an accompanying rash. Recognition of the bacterial origin of the illness allows one to practise prevention by isolating any infected persons; secondary prevention for contacts is possible by using prophylactic penicillin.

The dramatic reduction in the incidence of scarlet fever – in 1978, for instance, only 0.07 per cent of children aged 0 to 14 years in England and Wales had the illness[1] – is a good example of the way in which most infectious diseases affecting children have become less common and less severe since accurate records began to be kept, generally some time between 1850 and 1900. More important perhaps is the reduction in mortality from infectious diseases over the same period: it is the virtual elimination of death from infectious causes that has produced the greatest reduction of mortality in childhood. In 1870, for instance, the annual death rate of children under 15 from measles, whooping-cough, and diphtheria alone was 3250 per million.[2] By 1978, the death rate of children in the United Kingdom from *all* infective and parasitic causes, including pneumonia, meningitis and gastroenteritis, had dropped to 162 per million.[1] Most of the reduction in mortality from infectious diseases had, however, occurred before effective medical treatment and prevention were available. A striking example is that of measles: the annual death rate per million children had remained at about 1100 for several decades prior to 1915; it then declined rapidly, and was already virtually zero before immunization was introduced nationally in 1968.[2] Tuberculosis shows perhaps a more typical picture: the annual death rate per million population fell from approximately 3000 to just under 500 in the century before effective treatment with streptomycin first became available in 1948; the rate has since declined more rapidly and is now less than 50.

It is important to recognize the distinction between improvements in the health of children that have come about through specifically medical advances and those that are the result of less specific improvements such as better diet, the provision of clean water in abundance, and the proper disposal of waste and excreta. The undoubted successes in treating disease with the many new drugs that have become available in the last thirty years often encourage doctors to exaggerate the contribution that medical care has made to the health of developed countries such as the United Kingdom. Just as a disease like measles ceased to be a significant cause of death before the specific medical intervention of immunization became available, so also public health in general, as measured by life expectancy, had improved almost to present levels before the pharmacological revolution started. Over the last thirty years, life expectancy in this country has increased by four years, while in the previous sixty years it had increased by twenty-five years.[1]

The precise contribution made to overall standards of health in developed countries by 'public health' measures on the one hand, and medical care on the other has been well debated in recent years. Henry Miller[3] appeared to accept quite readily that the great improvement in public health owed little to the medical profession, while McKeown[2] amassed a considerable body of evidence to support this view. Dollery[4] concluded that McKeown's case in particular was overstated and pointed out that the purpose of medicine was to reduce morbidity as well as mortality. Beeson[5] went further by showing the degree of success that the medical profession has had in treating disease. He examined the recommended treatments for 362 diseases in the 1st (1927) and 14th (1975) editions of a standard textbook of medicine. He devised a scoring system for the recommended treatments that ranged from 1 – recommended treatment now regarded as valueless, to 10 – highly effective preventive treatment. In the 1927 edition, effective treatment or preventive measures (scoring 7 or 8) were available for 3 per cent of the diseases and highly effective measures (scoring 9 or 10) for a further 3 per cent. By 1975 these figures had risen to 28 and 22 per cent respectively.

There is no need to rehearse here the continuing arguments about the effectiveness of modern medical treatments. What is important to note is the complete unanimity between medical discussants in the debate about the sorts of medical research that are needed. Miller,[3] McKeown,[2] Dollery,[4] Beeson,[5] Burnet,[6] and Thomas[7] are all agreed that the major research efforts should be directed to basic biological science rather than to applied research into the treatment or palliation of specific conditions. 'The great need now, for the medicine of the future, is for more information at the most fundamental levels of the living process.'[7] Support for this belief has been provided by Comroe and Dripps,[8] in a paper refuting the idea, popular in US Government circles in the late 1960s and early 1970s, that research would be most cost-effective if directed only at particular diseases, and that basic, undirected research should not be supported. They enlisted the help of a large number of specialists in cardiovascular and pulmonary diseases in order to decide which had been the ten most important advances in that field in the previous thirty years. They then asked other specialists what had been the essential bodies of knowledge without which the ten most important advances could not have happened. They looked, for example, at electrocardiography, producing a chronological table showing the principal discoveries necessary before Einthoven produced his sensitive string galvanometer for measuring a human electrocardiogram in 1903, and the later discoveries that allowed others to develop his idea into modern electrocardiography. They listed 45 discoveries, ranging from the recognition by the ancient Greeks of early manifestations of electricity in living things such as fish or eels, through Galvani's observations of the contraction of heart muscle caused by electric discharge in 1791, to the recording of electrical activity of the bundle of His (part of the electrical control mechanism of the heart) from within the heart, via a cardiac catheter, by Scherlag in 1967. From each of the bodies of knowledge regarded as essential, Comroe and Dripps and their reviewers selected the key articles and examined them to see whether their authors had made any mention of any clinical intent in their research. Thirty-eight per cent of the key articles were not clinically orientated in any way, and could be said instead to have the goal of knowledge for the sake of knowledge.

From this brief examination of the nature of the medical enterprise three tentative conclusions may be drawn which will help to provide a perspective in which to place subsequent discussions of research on children, whether as a class of activity or as individual projects. First, it is evident from the examples given by Comroe and Dripps that research in a particular field usually involves the slow and painstaking accumulation of many separate pieces of information: electrocardiography did not suddenly burst upon the world; rather, it was the result of the gradual collection, over centuries, of items of knowledge in various scientific fields. Similarly, most research projects on children have relatively specific aims, the fulfilment of which represent minor rather than major advances in knowledge.

Secondly, the major advances in public health, measured in terms of reduced mortality and increased life expectancy, have not in general been the result of medical research or improved medical treatment or prevention. While medical research has sometimes led to the complete elucidation of the mechanism of a disease, it has more often led to what Thomas has described as 'halfway technology'.[9] He describes such technology as 'the kinds of things that must be done after the fact, in efforts to compensate for the incapacitating effects of certain diseases whose course one is unable to do very much about'. It is contrasted with 'non-technology' – the business of supportive therapy that is not directed at the mechanisms of disease – and full, or decisive, technology, which is not only direc-ted at the mechanism of a disease but depends on a full understanding of it. Examples of the latter are the prevention of haemolytic disease of the new-born, prevention of a variety of infectious diseases by immunization, and the treatment of endocrine disorders with appropriate hormones. Halfway technology, on the other hand, is concerned with activities such as renal dialysis or transplantation when renal failure has occurred, neonatal intensive care when a premature delivery has not been prevented, or the treatment of a cancer, after it has become established, by drugs or radiation. One notable feature of halfway technology is that it tends to be much more expensive and generally less effective than decisive technology.

The third point to be noted from the foregoing is the unanimity among many eminent commentators that priority should be given to basic biological research. Such research is usually necessary in order to achieve full understanding of the underlying mechanisms of disease, without which the 'decisive technology' described above cannot be developed. Some of the research projects that are carried out on children can be classified as basic research, in that they are designed in some way to clarify the mechanisms of disease, but many cannot, since they are aimed at improvements in 'halfway technology' or in supportive care.

The nature of research

The survey carried out amongst chairmen of research ethics committees and reported in Chapter 8 shows that approximately 500 clinical research projects on children are started each year in England and Wales. These projects cover the whole field of paediatrics and can be classified in many different ways. In the previous chapter, the possibility of classifying projects as either therapeutic or non-therapeutic was explored; later in the report, projects are classified according to the degree of risk they impose on child subjects. At this stage the intention is to describe the types of research undertaken in neutral terms so as to set the context for later discussion. A simple classification has been adopted, by the degree of physical intervention. The degree of physical intervention may vary from nothing to a very high level, when multiple and complex procedures are involved. In between lie the great majority of research interventions which require little to be done to the child subjects.

Examples of research activities involving no physical intervention might be the taking of case histories or simple observation. Both these activities have been important in accumulating data about the normal and abnormal development of many childhood skills. It has, for instance, been important to discover the ages at which normal children develop bladder control by day or by night so as to avoid the unnecessary use of various 'treatments' for nocturnal enuresis. Observation of the interactions between an infant or child and his mother may also be used: for example, a recent study[10] showed that mothers of very sick infants in a neonatal intensive care unit touched, smiled at, and looked face to face at their infants much less than the mothers of relatively well babies in the same unit. In some research projects observation may be supplemented by photography, as in a study of the changes in the 'dynamic tripod' grip used by children of various ages when holding a pencil.[11]

Amongst research projects requiring physical intervention, probably the most minor degree of intervention used at all frequently is the touching involved in measurements of various indices of size. Tanner and his associates, in particular, have measured thousands of children so as to produce charts showing the normal patterns of growth and the limits of normality at all ages and stages of childhood and adolescence. Some measurements are extremely simple, such as height, weight,[12] or head circumference; others are almost as simple physically, but potentially more upsetting emotionally, particularly the assessment of stages of puberty involving the examination of breasts, testes and penile growth, and the amount of pubic hair.[13,14] Some indices of growth require a greater degree of intervention, however, in order to establish reliable standard values. Measurement of the bone age of children, by taking an X-ray of one wrist and examining the extent of ossification of the bones thereof, provides useful information in a variety of growth disorders; standards could only be produced, however, by X-raying normal children.[15] A similar, more recent study used ultrasound examination to measure the size of the uterus and ovaries in a group of normal girls aged 7 to 17 years.[16] Standards were obtained showing the changes in volume of the uterus and ovaries that occur during puberty. That these might be useful in the diagnosis of girls thought to have abnormal puberty was then demonstrated by examining several girls with pathologically early or late puberty: those with early puberty had uteri and ovaries much larger than normal for their age and those with late puberty had organs much smaller than normal.

Many examples were given to the working group of research activities involving only a minor degree of physical intervention, and some will be mentioned here. It is likely that the most common of such activities is the taking of small amounts of additional blood for research purposes during venesections undertaken for therapeutic reasons. Collection of urine specimens is also common and may be required for many different reasons: an example was given to the working group of girls being asked to provide specimens of urine in a mobile laboratory that visited schools for a study of the prevalence of asymptomatic bacteriuria.[17] Other specimens may also be collected with little or nothing in the way of physical intervention. Two examples are the collection of milk teeth, after they have fallen out, for measurement of lead levels, and the taking of a few hairs from zinc-deficient children in order to see whether the zinc levels in hair and serum are related. Attachment of various machines to children may sometimes be of little consequence, but can also be quite upsetting to either the child subject or his parents. An example of the former would be the wearing of a specially adapted self-winding wrist watch that measures limb movement, as a child scratches, to assess the severity of eczema. On the other hand a technique called 'jugular venous plethysmography', although non-invasive and relatively safe, can by its appearance be quite upsetting. It is used to measure blood flow through the jugular veins of infants under various conditions and provides information about the amount of blood flowing through the brain and any changes in cranial volume.[18,19] It is generally performed on infants within a few days of birth; four strands of plastic tubing filled with mercury are tied firmly round the infant's head and connected to a transducer. Both internal jugular veins are then compressed by the investigator's fingers, stopping blood flow in the veins; the amount of blood in the infant's head rises so that the volume of the head also increases, stretching the strands of plastic tubing. The electrical resistance of the mercury in the tubing alters, and the alteration can be measured. However well an investigator explained this procedure beforehand, it is likely to be upsetting to some mothers to see their new babies' heads bound by this measuring device with the investigator's fingers pressing – albeit gently – into the babies' necks.

As one continues along the suggested scale, of the degree of physical intervention involved in a research procedure, it is apparent that blood sampling is far from being the only invasive procedure used. Every orifice of the human body has had instruments inserted during the course of research on children. Specially designed thermometers have been inserted into the ear or oesophagus; needles have been inserted through the ear-drum to sample the fluid, if any, in the middle ear cavity; tubes or endoscopes have been passed through the nose or mouth to all levels of the intestine from oesophagus to ileum, for pressure measurements, biopsy of the intestinal lining or sampling of intestinal fluid; similarly, tubes or endoscopes have been passed via the anus for investigation of the large bowel; catheters have been passed via the urethra into the bladder and beyond – into the ureters; and catheters have been passed into both veins and arteries, and sometimes inserted far enough to reach the heart.

Another sort of intervention is to give substances to the child subjects. These may be drugs for treatment purposes, substances for investigative purposes, or anaesthetics. An example of a project that not only illustrates the use of investigative substances but also the way in which many tests may be carried out on the same child subject, is given by Pullan and Hey's follow-up[20] of children ten years after they had been infected with respiratory syncytial virus in infancy. One hundred and thirty such children were tested, along with 111 other children who acted as controls. Each child took part in at least five tests, and some also had an additional blood test. Two of the tests measured various aspects of pulmonary function – in one case after vigorous exercise – and only involved breathing into various machines. The other three tests all involved the giving of substances. In one, the children breathed 100 per cent oxygen; in another, they breathed in histamine acid phosphate through a nebulizer until significant bronchospasm (the basic problem in asthma) occurred; and in the third, various substances were pricked into the skin to see whether an allergic response resulted. The giving of a substance for investigative purposes may also involve a greater degree of intervention, as in the assessment of a child's renal function. The latter is often expressed as the glomerular filtration rate, which is measured by observing how rapidly an inert substance is filtered out of the blood stream by the kidneys. The normal method for measuring the glomerular filtration rate is to set up an intravenous infusion through which the child is given a solution of an inert chemical called inulin until the concentration of inulin in the child's blood reaches a steady level. An example of the use of such a system is given by Berg and Johansson who investigated 61 girls aged 1½ to 15 years suffering from recurrent urinary tract infections and 13 controls of whom 7 were children in the age range 5 to 13 years.[21]

An example of the use of anaesthetics during investigations was given in the previous chapter.[22] The study involved rectal pressure measurements and rectal biopsies in children, some of whom – whether subjects or controls – had been anaesthetized for the purpose. More common than the use of anaesthetics, however, is the use of sedation while investigations are carried out on children. Suzuki *et al.*, for instance, wished to ascertain whether there was any difference between certain components of the acoustically evoked potentials in children and adults.[23] Acoustically evoked potentials are the electrical brain waves produced in response to a standard sound stimulus and detected by electrodes attached to various parts of the head. Suzuki *et al.* examined these potentials in 26 children considered to have normal hearing and aged from 1 to 7 years. They were tested either during natural sleep or under sedation induced by giving a sedative, triclofos, orally. The dose of triclofos given – 70 to 80 mg/kg body weight – was three times higher than that usually recommended.[24]

The third group of substances given to children are drugs given for therapeutic purposes. Trials of drugs – whether new, or ones that have previously been used in either children or adults – are probably less frequent than is commonly supposed. One indicator of this is provided by the journal *Archives of Disease in Childhood*. In 1983 it published 223 original articles and short reports, of which 9 were reports of drug trials, 5 were reports of various aspects of the pharmacology of particular drugs, and a few more were reports of uncommon side-effects of drugs. Of the nine drug trials, two reported comparisons of different methods of giving a drug already known to be effective, and two reported unsuccessful attempts to treat a condition, bronchiolitis, in which it was already suspected that the drugs would be ineffective. One paper reported a randomized controlled trial of indomethacin in the treatment of a neonatal heart condition, patent ductus arteriosus; the drug had been widely used in that condition for several years, but the authors wished to confirm that it was the drug, rather than changes in the infants' fluid balance, that was effective. Only four papers described the trial of drugs for particular groups of children in whom those drugs had not previously been used.

One area in which research projects have employed a high level of intervention has been in the treatment of acute lymphoblastic leukaemia. Not only have the drugs used been in general quite toxic, with high levels of side-effects, but they have in general been given intravenously or even intrathecally, i.e. by lumbar puncture. In addition, the central nervous system has often been irradiated with high doses of X-rays, and bone-marrow aspirations have been performed to follow the progress of the disease. The result of a continuing programme of trials of such therapies has, however, been a very great improvement in the prognosis for children with acute lymphoblastic leukaemia. These trials are a good example of the way in which, although individual research projects may only produce small improvements, a series of such projects may produce dramatic results. Another example of the latter effect would be the series of experiments that elucidated the cause, then improved the management and finally provided prevention of Rhesus haemolytic disease in new-born babies.

Future areas of research

While the foregoing classification of research according to the degree of intervention allows an overview of the sorts of things that are done to and with children, there are several other possible ways of classifying research. One such way is to look fairly broadly at the purposes of research: such a view may help to indicate the sorts of research on children that still need to be undertaken. Within the previous classification, there have been examples of projects attempting to define the normal, whether it be the normal age at which bladder control is developed, or the normal pattern of acoustically evoked potentials. Illingworth, in *The normal child*,[25] says that '. . . a thorough knowledge of the normal is an essential basis for the diagnosis of the abnormal'; few, if any, paediatricians would ever disagree with that statement. There are still areas in which little is known of the way in which normal children function, and so research to define the normal will continue.

Another group of projects were those designed to improve methods of investigation. There were examples such as an attempt to measure zinc levels in hair rather than blood, and the use of ultrasound in girls with abnormal puberty to measure the size of the uterus and ovaries. These are both examples of the way in which simpler, less invasive, and therefore, less distressing ways of investigating children are always being sought. The third group of projects described above were those concerned with improving therapy. Examples were only given of the use of drugs, but new therapies might also involve the use of hormones or blood products, physiotherapy, psychotherapy, or surgery, to mention but a few of the possibilities. Research into such therapies will obviously continue, but it is important to remember that it will often be the 'halfway technology' that was considered earlier in the chapter. In global terms, the major killing diseases in childhood are caused either by infections or by malnutrition. In developed countries such diseases are now uncommon, so that research tends to be directed to finding ways of treating or preventing life-threatening illnesses that each affect relatively few children, or non-life-threatening illnesses that may still affect many children.

There are three further groups of research projects that were not touched on in the classification by degree of intervention, but which are likely to become of increasing importance. First, there is the research necessary to elucidate basic disease mechanisms, without which one cannot progress from the 'halfway' technology described earlier to 'decisive' technology. Obviously, some of the information essential to such research is the measurement of normal factors and of how they are abnormal in children with specific diseases. But much, if not most, of the work of elucidating basic disease mechanisms will be carried out using *in vitro* techniques and, sometimes, animal models of the diseases. The need, therefore, for clinical research on children for this purpose is relatively limited. An example of the sort of disorder in which it would be extremely useful to discover basic disease mechanisms is obesity.

The second group of research projects that will become increasingly important includes projects designed to question established dogma. Reports of research that examines generally accepted routines in medical therapy do appear occasionally, and when they do, the results can be quite surprising. Watson *et al.*, for instance, undertook a reappraisal of routine bone marrow examinations carried out on children with acute lymphoblastic leukaemia or non-Hodgkin's lymphoma. Once remission has been induced in children with these diseases, it is usual for them to continue to receive maintenance chemotherapy for two to three years. Most protocols for maintenance chemotherapy, including those of the United Kingdom Acute Lymphoblastic Leukaemia trials organized by the Medical Research Council, have included the requirement of routine examination of the bone marrow at three-monthly intervals in order to detect early any signs of relapse. Watson and his colleagues carried out 557 such routine bone-marrow examinations, of which 9 showed evidence of relapse; only 2 of the 9 children had normal blood counts, however, while the remaining 7 had varying degrees of abnormality of their blood counts. Thus, the incidence of unexpected relapse was only 0.4 per cent, and Watson *et al.* were able to conclude that routine bone-marrow examinations during maintenance chemotherapy were not worthwhile. Unless performed under general anaesthetic, bone-marrow examination is traumatic for children, parents, and doctors, so that the findings of a project like this one can lead to a significant improvement in the care of children by obviating the need for an unnecessary procedure.

The third group of projects that are likely to become more common are those concerned with the provision of health care. The Black Report (*Inequalities in health*)[27] for instance, collected a large amount of information showing that after thirty years of the National Health Service there had been little or no reduction in social inequalities in health. Some of the findings are as follows:

'At birth and in the first month of life, twice as many babies of unskilled manual parents (class V) die as do babies of professional class parents (class I) and in the next 11 months 4 times as many girls and 5 times as many boys.'

'The extent of the problem may be illustrated by the fact that if the mortality rate of class I had applied to classes IV and V during 1970–72 . . . 74 000 lives of people aged under 75 would not have been lost. This estimate includes nearly 10 000 children.'

'For deaths caused by fire, falls and drowning the risk for boys (aged 1–14) in class V is 10 times the risk for their peers in class I. The corresponding ratio for deaths caused to youthful pedestrians by motor vehicles is more than 7:1.'

The Black Report showed that overall the mortality rate of boys aged 1 to 14 years in class V is more than double that of boys in class I, while the mortality rate of girls in class V is at least 1½ times that of girls in class I. Various recommendations were made, not only for strategies to try to reduce social inequalities, but also of areas in which further research was needed. The need for fuller reporting of accidents, for instance, is one that the Child Accident Prevention Trust is trying to meet.[28] Many other research projects will be needed, however, if one of the principal policy objectives of the Black Report – 'To give children a better start in life' – is to be capable of being fulfilled.

One area of the provision of health care that has been examined in recent years is perinatal mortality – stillbirths and deaths in the first week of life. In most developed countries the perinatal mortality rate has improved substantially over the last forty years. Many different factors have influenced the decline in perinatal mortality rates ranging from improvements in antenatal, and now even preconceptional, care to the greater availability of neonatal intensive care facilities. It has been suggested that the decline is primarily a reflection of improved social conditions with better care and nutrition in pregnancy. Non-specific factors such as these could be expected to exert their influence on the length of gestation and the rate of intrauterine growth, leading to improvements in birth weight. In fact, several studies in the United States, such as that of Williams and Chen,[29] have shown that improvements in birth weight account for only about one-fifth of the decline in perinatal mortality rates. The remaining four-fifths of the decline has been achieved by improvements in neonatal intensive care and the greater safety of caesarian section. A recent English paper also suggests that neonatal care has become quite effective. Wood conducted a confidential paediatric inquiry into neonatal deaths in the Wessex region in 1981 and 1982.[30] There were 386 neonatal deaths, at a rate of 5.8 per 1000 live births, of which 144 were due to lethal or severe malformations. Of the remaining 242 normally formed infants, factors operating before delivery accounted for 43 per cent of the deaths, factors after delivery for 33 per cent, and a combination of factors for the remaining 24 per cent. Adverse factors in medical care were identified in 38 deaths, 11 of these being due to errors in neonatal care. It was concluded that the greatest scope for improving the outcome of childbirth in Wessex lay in further advances in antenatal and obstetric care rather than in neonatal care. There appears to be good reason for suggesting that neonatal care is another area in which a whole variety of research projects has led to great improvements, just as has happened in the treatment of acute lymphoblastic leukaemia or the prevention of Rhesus haemolytic disease.

An area in which the provision of health care in Great Britain is inadequate at present is the immunization of children against infectious diseases. This has largely resulted from public fears about the safety of the vaccines used, and in particular about the safety of whooping-cough vaccine. New vaccines are constantly being developed and will continue to need to be tested on children. A recent American paper[31] described the successful trial of a new vaccine against chickenpox: the trial was successful in that there were few reactions to the vaccine all of which were minor, and the vaccine appeared to be completely effective. It seems likely that genetic engineering techniques will revolutionize the production of vaccines over the next decade, leading to many safer and more effective vaccines, but leading also to the need for them all to be tested on children.[32]

One cannot mention immunization without discussing, even if only in passing, the most serious problem in the provision of health care today. That is the problem of how to provide even the most simple level of health care for the hundreds of millions of children in developing countries. About seventeen million children under the age of 5 die each year around the world, fewer than one million of them coming from developed countries.[33] Thirteen million of these children die before the age of 1 year. Five million die of diarrhoea or gastroenteritis; between 3½ and 5 million die of infectious diseases for which immunizations with effectiveness greater than 80 per cent are available. Neonatal tetanus kills 1 million new-born babies each year: it may be prevented by giving women of child bearing age two doses of tetanus toxoid costing perhaps 15p. Whooping-cough kills at least half-a-million children, and perhaps many more. But the major killer, in association with malnutrition, is measles: the lowest estimate of annual childhood mortality is 1½ million worldwide, with some estimates as high as 3 million deaths. It can be prevented by a single dose of vaccine costing about 10p. If one's only concern were to save lives, a crude utilitarian analysis would always give the answer that the money spent on research on children in Great Britain would give a much quicker and greater return if it were spent on immunizing children in Third World countries. The United Nations declaration 'The rights of the child', adopted in 1959, includes principle 2: 'The child shall enjoy special protection and shall be given opportunities and facilities, by law and by other means, to enable him to develop physically, mentally, morally, spiritually and socially in a healthy and normal manner and in conditions of freedom and dignity. In the enactment of laws for this purpose the best interests of the child shall be the paramount consideration.'

Limitations and problems of research

To complete this attempt to provide an overview of research on children, it is necessary to consider some of its limitations and drawbacks. It is arguable that two of the most important medical discoveries this century (and they are perhaps the two most clinically important discoveries) were pure serendipity – simply chance observations. The first is well known – the sagacious observation by Fleming of the inhibitory effect of a mould on the growth of bacteria which led to the development of penicillin. The second is perhaps less well known: in the course of attempts to replace fluid loss in cholera victims in 1964, Phillips observed that while little or none of a salt and electrolyte solution given orally was absorbed, the addition of glucose to the solution resulted in most of it being absorbed.[34] This chance observation has formed the basis of oral rehydration therapy in diarrhoeal diseases: if information about this therapy could be spread universally, many of the 5 million deaths of children each year from such illness could be prevented.

Later in this report, risk will be discussed in some detail. It is important to realize that the harm, of which there is a certain risk in a given research project, may sometimes occur. One of the many improvements in neonatal care – contributing to the decline in perinatal mortality mentioned earlier – has been in the management of neonatal asphyxia. Soon after the Second World War it was found that administration of oxygen, *ad libitum,* to premature infants greatly improved their chances of survival when they developed respiratory problems such as hyaline membrane disease. A little later it was noted that many of the infants who survived were partially sighted or completely blind; they had a disorder, retrolental fibroplasia, that had hitherto been most uncommon. The probable link between high oxygen levels in the neonatal period and this sort of blindness was quickly recognized. Indeed, some physiologists would argue that information about the risks of high oxygen concentrations was already available before paediatricians started to give premature infants extra oxygen. Yet one group of investigators in the United States decided[35] that they should 'establish such a relationship (between high oxygen levels and retrolental fibroplasia) beyond question.'

They therefore allocated all infants weighing between 1000 and 1850 grams, and less than 12 hours old when admitted to their premature nursery, either to a high-oxygen therapy group receiving a mean of 69 per cent oxygen, or to a low-oxygen therapy group receiving just enough oxygen to abolish cyanosis. There was no significant difference in mortality between the groups. Of 36 infants in the high-oxygen group, 8 had severe retrolental fibroplasia causing permanent blindness, and 22 had a milder form of the disorder. None of the 28 infants in the low-oxygen group had severe damage and only 2 had the milder form of the disorder.

The investigators had therefore established to their satisfaction that high levels of oxygen caused a blinding condition in new-born infants. But in the process they had also managed to raise many ethical problems, some of which will be mentioned here. Pappworth, in *Human guinea pigs,*[36] raises the question of whether the study was necessary at all. He cites four reports, published before this particular trial was likely to have started, which one could reasonably expect the investigators to have read; all of them provide strong evidence for the link between high oxygen levels and retrolental fibroplasia. The ethics of undertaking a controlled trial of which the end-point to be sought is a blinding condition have also been discussed frequently. Approval has been voiced only by those who think that only scientific certainty that is statistically verifiable is of value in determining medical therapy. The role conflict to which such attitudes may lead in doctors – i.e. the conflict between the degree of certainty that a doctor *qua* scientist seeks, compared to the degree of certainty with which a doctor *qua* physician is likely to be satisfied – has been discussed in a recent editorial in the *Journal of Medical Ethics.*[37]. It is important to realize, however, that the analysis of the study described above was statistically inept and in parts incorrect. Several miscalculations led the authors to give their results a lower degree of statistical significance than was in fact the case. More importantly though, there appears to have been no attempt to analyse the results sequentially, i.e. as they were obtained. Had this been done, it is certain that a highly significant difference, statistically, between the two groups of infants would have been obtained when many fewer infants had been enrolled in the trial. If one compares those infants with signs of retrolental fibroplasia – whether mild or severe – to those with no such signs, statistical analysis shows that there is less than one chance in a million that the results could have been obtained by accident. In medicine, one is usually satisfied that a causal relationship has been demonstrated if there is less than one chance in a hundred that it happened by accident. If in this study only half as many infants had been used, it is almost certain that a highly significant result would have been obtained. Indeed, if only 16 infants had been used, instead of 64, and the outcome for these 16 had been distributed in the same way as for the whole group of 64, then a statistically significant result would still have been obtained. In other words, even though this study was only undertaken for the purposes of scientific certainty, the science was done badly, and many infants had their sight damaged unnecessarily even for the scientific purpose.

The study of retrolental fibroplasia has been examined at length because of the ethical problems it raises. They demonstrate certain questions that need to be asked of any proposed research project on children:

Is it necessary?
Does it use appropriate methods to test the hypothesis suggested?
Are the risks to the subjects acceptable?
Is the proposed statistical analysis competent?

Perhaps the most obvious limitation of research on children is that research projects may produce no useful results, even if they do not produce any harm. Even whole series of research projects may produce little useful information. The mortality from asthma in children in this country, for example, has shown no significant decrease in the last twenty-five years. Indeed, in the early 1960s, mortality from asthma in children aged 5 to 14 years rose very steeply, before settling back to approximately the earlier level by the early 1970s.[38] Similarly, although the treatment of diabetes mellitus has shown considerable improvement since the discovery of insulin about sixty years ago, scientists appear to be little closer to being able to prevent it.

One example of the role conflict in which doctors may find themselves was given earlier. Another sort of role conflict may also arise in the setting of research on children. The practicalities of developing a career by publishing papers, that either report observations on children or the results of research projects on children, may act against the best interests of the child subjects by encouraging a doctor either consciously or unconsciously to inflate the possible benefit or to increase the risks of a research project.

There is an incentive for doctors to carry out research in order to improve their career prospects rather than to improve the health of children. Barber, in a large survey of medical researchers in the United States, showed one result of the competitiveness that is inherent in medical research: 'researchers who did not do well in the scientific or in the local-institutional competition for rewards were more likely than others to be involved in studies with less favourable risk/benefits ratios for subjects.'[39] Investigators might perhaps bear in mind Bernard Shaw's comment in the preface to *The Doctor's Dilemma*: 'The right to knowledge is not the only right; and its exercise must be limited by respect for other rights, and for its own exercise by others.'

Non-medical research

The purpose of this chapter has been not only to give an impression of the sorts of things that are done to and with children during clinical research, but also to provide a wider perspective within which to assess such research. One element of such a perspective remains to be considered: the non-medical activities, and in particular non-medical research, in which children may become involved. Some non-medical research may be closely related – studies, for instance, by dentists in the prevention or treatment of dental caries. In the United Kingdom, many such studies would be submitted to a local research ethics committee for approval, but not all dentists would be under any sort of obligation to make such a submission. There are often close links between medical and nursing research, but the latter is seldom submitted to independent review. An exception to the rule, however, is a study of increased parental care for children in hospital now being undertaken in Cardiff: both the medical and the nursing elements of this study were submitted independently for ethical review. Much nursing research is sociological in nature, looking at the effectiveness of nurses as health educators, for instance, or examining methods of preparing children for hospital admission, with follow-up studies of their reactions to hospital. Another example of nursing research given to the working group – but actually carried out several years ago – was of a trial of sheepskins in the prevention of bedsores. They were placed under half the patients on a ward, and not under the rest: the trial continued even when early results showed the sheepskins to be very useful.

Other areas in which research is undertaken on children include psychology, sociology, education, and social welfare. When psychological research is carried out by psychologists based in a hospital, proposals for research projects will generally be subject to ethical review by the local research ethics committee. If the research is undertaken in a school, the controls are likely to be fewer. There are some exceptions to this general picture. All researchers, of whatever profession, who wish to carry out research in schools run by the Inner London Education Authority have to obtain prior approval from the ILEA Research and Statistics Department as well as the Education Committee. Control of educational research in other areas of the country is variable, though usually major projects will require approval from the Local Authority Education Committee. It appears, however, that educational experiment may not infrequently be undertaken without parental involvement or consent. The working group was told, for instance, by one of its members of a London borough in which the intake to a primary school a few years ago had been divided at random into two sections. One section was taught to read using the normal alphabet, while the other was taught with the Initial Teaching Alphabet. There had been no prior discussion with or consent from the parents, yet there was a risk of delaying the development of reading ability in some of the children and, therefore, the development of their overall intellectual abilities.

Further examples can be given of projects carried out with children in school that were not specifically concerned with education, but which appeared to have an element of using children in school as a readily available study population. Elphick,[40] for instance, wished to compare two methods of testing children's abilities to lip-read: in one method he mouthed words and sentences to the child subjects, without giving any auditory clues, while in the other, a video-recording was played of him saying the same words and sentences, but without any sound output. The subjects were twenty 9-year-old primary school children. Although thanks are given to the headmaster and children of the primary school concerned, there is no mention of parental consent or ethics committee approval. Haggard *et al.* report[41] on a two-part study in which they were examining a new method for screening hearing ability in school children in order to try to improve the selectivity of current methods. School screening hearing tests are generally performed in the absence of specific parental permission while children are at school; parents may only be informed of the result if it is abnormal. In the first part of this study, 134 children aged about 5 years old were tested by speech audiometry. In the second part, 228 children between 5 and 6 years were tested in a soundproof booth in a specially equipped van using three tests, speech audiometry, pure tone audiometry, and impedance tympanometry: routine school screening of hearing usually employs one, or at most, two of these tests. As in the previous example, there is no mention of parental consent or ethics committee approval being obtained, though this may be an omission in both examples; nor is there any suggestion either that parents were ever present or were invited to be present during the testing.

Another example of school-based research tends to reinforce the impression that parents generally are not involved in such research projects. FitzHerbert reports a project financed by the Social Science Research Council the aim of which was to 'develop an integrated preventive child care system focussed on primary schools'.[42] Primary school teachers periodically screened a group of 200 9- and 10-year-old children for 'lack of confidence, temper tantrums, non-attendance at school, extreme withdrawal, attention seeking, and incontinence', in order 'to identify children at risk of delinquency, habitual truancy, maladjustment or educational failure'. Initially, 28 children, and finally 59 children, were so identified. It had been hoped that individual preventive action could be undertaken for each 'child in need' by various members of social, school psychological, educational social work, child guidance, or child health, services. 'However, resources were too meagre for case work intervention on a significant scale, and many of the cases identified were not sufficiently "bad" to justify "interference" by a team member in the affairs of a family which had not asked for help.' Instead, activity groups were set up to which the identified children went for weekly sessions of 1½ hours after school. Eight children were in each group, with a group leader and another helper; 'none of the leaders had any training in group work with children' and most were either volunteers or social work students on placement. Although it is concluded that the activity groups are a 'promising technique', no attempt at objective assessment was made. Parents are mentioned only twice in the report. Describing one child from 'a chronic anti-school family' whose behaviour improved during the project, the report says: 'When next absent, her mother (previously only abusive in response to attendance queries) sent a note.' The other mention of parents is found amid 'five useful principles for activity group organisation': 'Collecting and taking children home individually provides a useful opportunity for one-to-one chats, as well as minimal friendly contact with parents.' There does not otherwise appear to have been any attempt to involve parents; there is no suggestion that any attempt was made to explain the project to parents or to gain their consent for their children's participation; there is no mention that the change in the method of carrying out the project was discussed with the funding agency or with anyone else who might have provided peer review.

No startling conclusions can be drawn from the few examples given of non-medical research; but it does appear that problems similar to those found in medical research, such as parental involvement, parental consent, and the potential degree of emotional upset caused to children by a project, may occur. The model of peer review provided by research ethics committees in the health services does appear to be one that could usefully be applied by educational authorities. It would appear that research on children in both the medical and the non-medical spheres may be of more limited value than its protagonists would wish to admit.

References

1. Forfar, J. O. Demography, vital statistics and the pattern of disease in childhood. In *Textbook of paediatrics* (3rd edn) (eds. J. O. Forfar and G. C. Arneil) pp.1–25. Churchill Livingstone, Edinburgh (1984).
2. McKeown, T. *The role of medicine,* pp.91–106. Blackwell, Oxford (1979).
3. Miller, H. *Medicine and society,* pp.1–16. Oxford University Press (1973).
4. Dollery, C. *The end of an age of optimism,* pp.14–16. Nuffield Provincial Hospitals Trust, London (1978).
5. Beeson, P. B. Changes in medical therapy during the past half century. *Medicine* **59**(2), 79–99 (1980).
6. Burnet, M. Biomedical Research: Changes and Opportunities. *Perspect. Biol. Med.* **24,** 511–24 (1981).
7. Thomas, L. Medical lessons from history. In *The medusa and the snail,* pp.158–75. Allen Lane, London (1980).
8. Comroe, J. H., and Dripps, R. D. Scientific basis for the support of biomedical science. *Science* **192,** 105–11 (1976).
9. Thomas, L. The technology of medicine. In *The lives of a cell,* pp.31–6. Allen Lane, London (1980).

10. Minde, K., Whitelaw, A., Brown, J., and Fitzhardinge, P. Effect of neonatal complications in premature infants on early parent-infant interactions. *Devl Med. & Child Neurol.* **25**, 763–777 (1983).

11. Ziviani, J. Qualitative changes in dynamic tripod grip between seven and fourteen years of age. *Devl Med. & Child Neurol.* **25**, 778–82 (1983).

12. Tanner, J. M., Whitehouse, R. H., and Takaishi, M. Standards from birth to maturity for height, weight, height velocity and weight velocity: British children, 1965. *Archs Dis. Childh.* **41**, 454–71 and 613–35 (1966).

13. Marshall, W. A. and Tanner, J. M. Variations in the pattern of pubertal changes in girls. *Archs Dis. Childh.* **44**, 291–303 (1969).

14. —— and ——. Variations in the pattern of pubertal changes in boys. *Archs Dis. Childh.* **45**, 13–23 (1970).

15. Tanner, J. M., Whitehouse, R. H., and Healey, M. J. R. *A new system for estimating skeletal maturity from the hand and wrist, with standards derived from a study of 2,600 healthy British children.* International Children's Centre, Paris (1962).

16. Ivarrson, S-A., Nilsson, K. O., and Persson, P-H. Ultrasonography of the pelvic organs in prepubertal and postpubertal girls. *Archs Dis. Childh.* **58**, 352–4 (1983).

17. Asscher, A. W., McLachlan, M. S. F., Verrier Jones, R., Meller, S., Sussman, M., Harrison, S., Johnston, H. H., Sleight, G., and Fletcher, E. W. Screening for asymptomatic urinary-tract infection in schoolgirls. *Lancet* **ii**, 1–4 (1973).

18. Dear, P. R. F. Effect of feeding on jugular venous blood flow in the normal newborn infant. *Archs Dis. Childh.* **55**, 365–70 (1980).

19. Milligan, D. W. A. Positive pressure ventilation and cranial volume in newborn infants. *Archs Dis. Childh.* **56**, 331–5 (1981).

20. Pullan, C. R., and Hey, E. N. Wheezing, asthma and pulmonary dysfunction 10 years after infection with respiratory syncytial virus in infancy. *Br. med. J.* **284**, 1665–9 (1982).

21. Berg, U. B., and Johansson, S. B. Age as a main determinant of renal functional damage in urinary tract infection. *Archs Dis. Childh.* **58**, 963–9 (1983).

22. Molnar, D., Taitz, L. S., Urwin, O. M., and Wales, J. K. H. Anorectal manometry results in defecation disorders. *Archs Dis. Childh.* **58**, 257–61 (1983).

23. Suzuki, T., Hirabayashi, M., and Kobayashi, K. Auditory middle responses in young children. *Br. J. Audiol.* **17**, 5–9 (1983).

24. *British National Formulary No. 7.* British Medical Association and The Pharmaceutical Society of Great Britain, London (1984).

25. Illingworth, R. S. *The normal child* (8th edn) p.2. Churchill Livingstone, Edinburgh (1983).

26. Watson, D. K., Robinson, A. E., and Bailey, C. C. A reappraisal of routine marrow examination therapy of acute lymphoblastic leukaemia. *Archs Dis. Childh.* **56**, 392–4 (1981).

27. Working Group on Inequalities in Health (Chairman: Sir D. Black). *Report: Inequalities in health.* DHSS, London (1980).

28. Jackson, R. H. and Gaffin, J. The Child Accident Prevention Trust. *Archs Dis., Childh.* **58**, 1031–3 (1983).
29. Williams, R. L. and Chen, P. M. Identifying the sources of the recent decline in perinatal mortality rates in California. *New Engl. J. Med.* **306**, 207–14 (1982).
30. Wood, B., Catford, J. C., and Cogswell, J. J. Confidential paediatric inquiry into neonatal deaths in Wessex, 1981 and 1982. *Br. med. J.* **288**, 1206–8 (1984).
31. Weibel, R. E., Neff, B. J., Kuter, B. J., Guess, H. A., Rothenberger, C. A., Fitzgerald, A. J., Connor, K. A., McLean, A. A., Hilleman, M. R., Buynak, E. B., and Scolnick, E. M. Live attenuated varicella virus vaccine: efficacy trial in healthy children. *New Engl. J. Med.* **310**, 1409–15 (1984).
32. Young, C. R. Editorial: Towards new vaccines. *J. R. Soc. Med.* **77**, 261–3 (1984).
33. Rohde, J. E. Why the other half dies: the science and politics of child mortality in the Third World. *Assignment children (UNICEF, Geneva)* **61/62**, 35–67 (1983).
34. Phillips, R. A. Water and electrolyte losses in cholera. *Fed. proc. Fedn Am. Socs exp. Biol.* **23**, 705–12 (1964).
35. Lanman, J. T., Guy, L. P., and Dancis, J. Retrolental fibroplasia and oxygen therapy. *J. Am. Med. Assoc.* **155**, 223–6 (1954).
36. Pappworth, M. H. *Human guinea pigs,* pp.221–2. Routledge & Kegan Paul, London (1967).
37. Editorial. Ethics, philosophy and clinical trials. *J. med. Ethics* **9**, 59–60 (1983).
38. Colley, J. R. T. The epidemiology of respiratory disease in childhood. In *Recent advances in paediatrics,* vol. 5 (ed. D. Hull) pp.221–58. Churchill Livingstone, Edinburgh (1976).
39. Barber, B., Lally, J. J., Makarushka, J. L., and Sullivan, D. *Research on human subjects: problems of social control in medical experimentation,* p. x. Transaction Books, New Brunswick, NJ (1979).
40. Elphick, R. Comparison of live and video presentation of a speech reading test with children. *Br. J. Audiol.* **18**, 109–15 (1984).
41. Haggard, M. P., Wood, E. J., and Carroll, S. Speech, admittance and tone tests in school screening, reconciling economics with pathology and disability perspectives. *Br. J. Audiol.* **18**, 133–53 (1984).
42. FitzHerbert, K. Therapeutic groups for children. *Concern* (National Children's Bureau, London) **47**, 22–6 (1983).

4

The structure of the argument

Our task in this report is not merely to make recommendations but to give reasons for them. It is therefore necessary to offer some account of how we think one can argue for conclusions in this field. Since the conclusions are about what ought or ought not to be done or permitted, the arguments will be moral or ethical arguments; and the discipline which assesses such arguments is moral philosophy, or ethics in the narrow philosophical sense. As we shall see, however, the two main approaches to moral argument which have been advocated by philosophers are, both of them, more sophisticated versions of ways of thinking which suggest themselves quite naturally to non-philosophers when they have to think about moral questions. This is in part because the thinking of ordinary people has been deeply, if unconsciously, influenced by what philosophers have said in the past; but more because those philosophers themselves were making explicit certain tendencies which were already there in everyday thinking. Our problem will be to find a way of combining both these approaches in a consistent procedure which could be used by, say, an ethics committee when considering a particular research project. But first we must explain each approach separately.

The first approach bases itself on rights and duties. Most of us think that people have rights which it is the duty of other people to respect. We also think that there are other duties besides the duty to respect people's rights. In our present field we need not look far for examples. If we think of any doctor and any patient of his, we shall be in no doubt that the doctor has the duty to do what he can to cure or alleviate the patient's trouble; not to cause harm to the patient unless that is required for the purpose of achieving some greater good for him, and then only with his consent; not to use his professional relationship to secure for himself advantages which lie outside the implied contract with his patient (for example, he may rightly expect to be paid for his services, but ought not to seek to obtain sexual favours or a place in the patient's will); not to divulge information given in confidence; and so on. These duties are commonly expressed in another way, by saying that the patient has a right to have or not to have this or that done to him.

In a research project the subject is sometimes the patient of the researcher and sometimes not. If he is, then all the above duties will be held to apply, and there may be a conflict between them and the furtherance of the research. If he is not, some of these duties may be absent (for example, the researcher has no duty to try to cure the subject) but those duties will remain which anybody, whether he is a doctor or not, owes to his fellow human beings: for example, not to subject him to physical interventions without his consent; not to lie to him, or make promises that he is not going to fulfil.

The researcher may also think that he has, as a scientist, other duties not so far mentioned. In becoming a scientist, he has dedicated himself to the increase of knowledge, and thus to the duty of pursuing the truth even at considerable cost to himself. If he is a medical scientist, it will not be merely truth for truth's sake that he is pursuing; he will be inspired by the hope that his discoveries may benefit mankind by making possible new therapies, and he will think that this lays on him a duty to make every effort to further his research. This applies to many other kinds of scientist – indeed, to any researcher; for example, a physiologist or a psychologist or a chemist or an engineer – whose discoveries might be of practical use. It is easy to see how in clinical research this duty can conflict with others that we have mentioned. For example, an intervention which is necessary for the research may risk harming the subject without hope of any compensating benefit to him.

Rights and duties are the main preoccupation of the so-called deontological school of moral philosophers. They usually base themselves on the common moral convictions that most of us have, using them as data in much the same way as empirical science uses the facts of observation. In the words of Sir David Ross, 'The moral convictions of thoughtful and well-educated people are the data of ethics just as sense-perceptions are the data of a natural science. Just as some of the latter have to be rejected as illusory, so have some of the former; but as the latter are rejected only when they are in conflict with other more accurate sense-perceptions, the former are rejected only when they are in conflict with other convictions which stand better the test of reflection.'[1] The method employed is thus intuitive: it consists in an appeal to moral intuition of a sort that can dispense with argument. As H. A. Prichard, one of the leaders of the school, said, 'If we do doubt whether there is really an obligation to originate *A* in a situation *B*, the remedy lies not in any process of general thinking, but in getting face to face with a particular instance of the situation *B,* and then directly appreciating the obligation to originate *A* in that situation.'[2]

As well as being intuitionists, such philosophers are usually pluralists: they claim to find in our common moral convictions a plurality of principles which cannot be reduced to one another or to some higher single principle. Thus, the duty not to interfere with other people's bodies is a different principle from the duty not to deceive them, and both are different from the duty to be just in apportioning punishments and rewards. These duties are independent of one another and independently recognized. Most deontologists, however, try to reduce their principles to a manageable number – a list of duties from which the rest can be derived. Among those relevant to our enquiry we may mention duties of beneficence and non-maleficence; the duty to act justly or fairly; and the duty not to deceive. Virtues and principles of these four kinds are made the basis of his moral system by G. J. Warnock, who, however, gives as his reason for commending them that their recognition would 'work towards amelioration of the human predicament'.[3] This is in substance a utilitarian reason and therefore would bring him within the scope of the second approach to be considered below, although he does not call himself a utilitarian.

Besides these principles which apply generally to everybody, there are also thought to be particular duties which attach to certain roles. We have already mentioned the doctor's particular duty to his own patients to promote their health and respect their confidences, and the scientist's duty to pursue the truth. And, as we have seen, to some of these duties there correspond rights: thus the patient has a right that his doctor should give promotion of the patient's health priority over the interests of other people who might eventually be benefited by discoveries made in the course of research on the patient; and those who are paying the scientist have a right that he should pursue his research (indeed, this will often be in his contract of employment).

This kind of deontology or pluralistic intuitionism is tailored to fit the convictions of ordinary people; and consequently it accords so well with them that it has with good reason been called 'the moral philosophy of the man in the street'. However, it does face certain difficulties, to which we shall return. If the duties it lays on us are treated as absolute and admitting of no exceptions, there will be a problem of what we ought to do if they conflict in particular cases, as they seem often to do. On the other hand, if they are treated as only prima-facie obligations (Ross's term), any of which can be overridden by another in cases of conflict, then an account has still to be given of how to decide which is to override which. Usually, deontologists at this point make a further appeal to intuition to settle the conflict: one of the duties will be perceived on reflection as more stringent than the other. But if a doctor who is also a researcher is in doubt whether he may properly take a blood sample at some small risk to his patient in order to further an important piece of research, his intuitions may not give a firm answer, and different people's intuitions may give different answers.

There is also the general problem of how we should justify the moral convictions on which we are to place so much weight. In the past, people have had some moral convictions which most of us would now repudiate, such as the conviction that wives ought to obey their husbands in all things. And at the present time, if children say that the sexual morality of their parents is a set of irrational taboos, can the parents quash this objection by appealing to their own moral convictions? Our common moral convictions may be sound, but it would be good to have a way of showing why they are.

In contrast to this deontological approach via rights and duties, we find in the literature, alongside it, much said about calculations of the risks and benefits attached to particular pieces of research. The idea is that if the benefits likely to be achieved (either to the patient, or to our knowledge of his disorder, or to medical science in general) are greater than the risks incurred, then the research is justified. The whole of Chapter 5 below is devoted to the discussion of how to assess risks, and of how to decide which are justified.

This kind of calculation is often called risk/benefit or cost/benefit analysis, and is used in many fields. It is, as we shall see, far from being generally accepted as a safe way of making moral decisions. But, like the deontological approach, it has a natural appeal. What could be more obvious, it might be said, than that we ought, when engaging in any activity involving risk to ourselves and our fellow men and women, to balance the risks against the likelihood of benefit, not incurring any risk that is not justified by the benefits to be expected. In more technical language, and in fields such as economics where it is thought that the risks and benefits can at least in theory be quantified, it is said that the product of the probability of an outcome and its utility (positive or negative) should be taken as its 'expected utility', and that action chosen which maximizes the 'expectation of utility', i.e. the sum of those products over all possible outcomes of an action.

This is in accord with a simple version (too simple to be acceptable) of the philosophical position known as utilitarianism. Positive and negative utility (benefit and harm) are now commonly defined in terms, not of pleasure or even happiness, as the classical utilitarians often did, but of preference-satisfaction.[4] It is important, however, to specify *who* expects the utility or disutility (hopes for the benefit or faces the risk of harm). A completely selfish risk/benefit analysis might be done by an individual purely in his own interest. Or someone (for example, a doctor) might do such an analysis purely in the interest of another individual (his patient). Suppose, for instance, that he balances the risk of death from an operation against the hope of a complete recovery. Only probabilities of benefits and harm to that individual will then be considered. Groups as well as individuals can reason in this way: such, perhaps, were the strategic analyses done by the American forces in Vietnam, which were concerned only with benefits to American policy, not to the Vietcong.

On the other hand, there could be a completely impartial risk/ benefit analysis in which the risk of harm or the benefit to *anybody* counted equally. It is the second, impartial kind of analysis which utilitarianism prescribes. It has, indeed, been attacked on precisely this ground, that it bids a doctor treat his professional duty to his own patients as of no greater weight than benefits he might confer on all and sundry by his researches.

This is only one example of a kind of criticism of utilitarianism which has been extremely common and has seemed conclusive to many. It proceeds by bringing utilitarianism into conflict with common moral convictions (the same as form the basis of deontological systems). Cases are adduced in which a utilitarian, seeking to maximize the expectation of utility, would have not merely to condone but to prescribe actions which most people would agree to be manifestly wrong. A common example in the literature is that of the surgeon who arranges to waylay and murder an innocent person, extracts his kidneys and other organs, and transplants them into his own patients, thereby saving several lives at the expense of one. Such a course, it is said, should be prescribed by a utilitarian, because the benefit to the greater, number outweighs the cost to the one. The same might be said if the victim, instead of being quarried for transplants, were made the subject of scientifically useful experiments which benefited mankind in general. Most such criticisms rely on the rights of people which everybody recognizes, not to have this kind of thing done to them, and on our duty to respect such rights.

There has thus seemed to be a tension between utilitarian thinking, with its risk/benefit analyses and its stress on the consequences of actions and on impartiality between the interests of everybody, and deontological thinking, with its appeals to rights and duties irrespective of consequences, and to duties to particular people in accordance with those people's rights, which are not owed to others. Yet both approaches have a firm basis in our ordinary moral thinking: we do attach importance to risks and benefits, and we do treat certain rights as sacrosanct, quite regardless of the benefits to be secured by infractions of them.

It is important to notice that this tension exists even *within* deontology, if it admits duties of beneficence and non-maleficence. These duties are, indeed, a kind of fragment of utilitarianism inside deontology, and conflicts can arise as well between them and the deontologist's other principles as between deontology and utilitarianism as a whole. These moral conflicts are at the centre of the dispute between the schools, and our working group has had to consider whether there could be any way of reconciling the two approaches in a practical procedure for addressing them which would retain the insights of both.

One way that has been suggested is to treat certain entrenched rights as side-constraints upon our utilitarian calculations, or, as R. M. Dworkin puts it, as 'trumps'.[5] That is to say, if to do the best for all considered impartially would involve infringing one of these rights, the rights are to prevail. That, it is suggested, is why we are not to commit murder however great the balance of benefits over costs. Although in that case the suggestion is attractive, it does not overcome all the difficulties. It does not tell us how to decide *which* rights ought to be entrenched in this way. And it does not allow us to say, as we may often want to say, that some rights can be overridden when great disasters will ensue if they are respected, but that lesser benefits will not justify their infringement. An example is where we undoubtedly infringe people's rights to liberty by confining them in quarantine in order to control epidemics. In the field of our present enquiry, shall we not want to say that some relatively minor interventions, which everybody would think justified if the benefits to medical science were enormous, would be unjustified if the benefits were small or uncertain? But the black-and-white character of the 'trumps' theory does not allow it to make such distinctions.

A more sophisticated suggestion relies on the separation of moral or ethical thinking into at least two levels. At the practical level at which most of us operate for most of the time, what the deontologists and pluralists and intuitionists say is largely correct. We do have a plurality of intuitive principles, many of them concerned with people's rights and duties, and we do treat these principles as having great authority. We react instantly and with strong repugnance to proposed breaches of them by ourselves or others; for practical purposes we treat some of them as sacrosanct, and all as of dominant importance. Many are enshrined in codes of ethics and lists of human rights. And it is a good thing that we think like this, because if we allowed ourselves to carry out elaborate risk/benefit analyses on particular occasions, we should nearly always get them wrong, either from a human inability to predict the consequences of our actions, or from an equally human tendency to deceive ourselves about the probabilities of benefit and harm. A researcher may convince himself that he will revolutionize the treatment of cancer by carrying out some questionable experiment, when his more judicious and less involved colleagues could tell him that the risks were much greater than he thinks and the likelihood of a major breakthrough very small. That is why we have ethics committees to sanction research projects, and why they should have firm guidelines such as we shall propose.

However, though it is right that we should think like deontologists in the normal course of our life and practice, it may be suggested that something has been left out of the account. Intuitive thinking is, as we have seen, not self-sustaining. We need a way of deciding what principles we should entrench, what intuitions we should cultivate, and what to do when they conflict. What is to be the content of the education of the 'thoughtful and well-educated people' who are Ross's court of appeal (see above)? When people are training to be doctors, or becoming researchers, what ought their seniors to say to them? And how are they to know whether their seniors are giving the best advice, when so much in medicine is changing that different principles may be appropriate to new conditions? To cope with this problem, it is suggested that a higher, 'critical', level of thinking is needed, by which we can criticize the principles and intuitions used at the lower level, and adjudicate between them in particular conflicts.

This higher level, it is suggested, is utilitarian. We should have, and teach, and cultivate in ourselves, those intuitions and those intuitive principles whose general acceptance in the profession and outside it will do the best, all in all, for those affected, considered impartially. (For discussion of this proposal, see Griffin, *op.cit.*)[4] The advocates of this view will often go on to say that nearly all the traditional principles and rights, including those mentioned earlier, could be justified, in general, by this kind of thinking. It *is* for the best, for example, that doctors should acknowledge special duties to their own patients, including the duty to respect their privacy and bodily integrity, unless the patients consent to invasions of them. If people, and doctors in particular, were not brought up to respect these principles, much more harm than good would result in the field of health care.

It will, however, sometimes happen, as we have seen, that sound general principles conflict with one another in particular cases. Most people would agree that research leading to the advancement of medical knowledge ought not to be hampered. And most people would agree that patients and other subjects have a right not to be experimented on without their consent. Deontologists may say that these common convictions need no justification. Utilitarians will say that they can be justified by the obvious utility of accepting them. We do not need much imagination to see the harm that would come of allowing researchers to shanghai people against their will and cut them up: confidence in the medical profession would be diminished, to put it mildly. And yet the benefits of increased medical knowledge are immense. So what is an ethics committee, to which a particular research project is submitted for approval, to do when, if it blesses a project, patients' rights will be infringed, but if it does not, important and useful research will be inhibited? This dilemma confronts us even when the proposed research subjects are adults; with children there are, as we shall see, further complications.

To some extent these problems can be coped with in advance by adopting general guidelines which attempt to hold a balance between the principles. Our enquiry will suggest guidelines of this sort. We shall assume, for example, that the requirement of consent to an experiment should be treated as sacrosanct in the case of competent adult subjects, because of the harm that would come of any weakening of this principle, the discussion and justification of which is outside our terms of reference. And, in extending the principle to children, we shall propose that proxy consent by parents or guardians should be allowable, subject to severe restrictions on the extent of the risks to which children may be thus submitted.

In determining the precise degree of risk, those of different philosophical persuasions will proceed differently. If we think that our common convictions need no justification, we shall appeal to general consensus, among those who have reflected on the problem, that that is the limit of acceptable risk. If, on the other hand, we either cannot find any such consensus, or do not regard mere consensus as enough of an argument (because people might come to think differently) we shall seek deeper foundations for the same practical prescriptions by pointing out the evil consequences that would result if the limits were put higher, or lower, than we propose. If they are put lower, then research which could be of value will be stopped in order to preserve the rights of children in cases where the preservation of those rights would make a negligible difference to the children's welfare or safety. To use the same example as before: the taking of small blood samples by pricking children's fingers, with consent of their parents and assent by the children, might be forbidden, even if the research project were likely to be of appreciable value. On the other hand, if the limits were put higher, then there would be danger that potentially quite harmful experiments would be allowed just because researchers with gleams in their eyes had prevailed on parents who did not fully understand what was being proposed, or upon gullible or perfunctory or complaisant ethics committees.

A case we have already mentioned illustrates the type of decision that may face us in framing or applying guidelines. A researcher asks to be allowed to perform a renal biopsy for research purposes on a child who is undergoing an abdominal operation. We have expressed the opinion (Chapter 1, pp.10–11)

that the risk from this is more than negligible. Should it nevertheless be permitted if very great benefits are expected from the
research? In the example reported we doubt whether this was so.
We have similar doubts whether it would ever be the case in
practice that the benefits justified the risk. We think that the
likelihood that *both* the benefits would be very great *and* there
would be no other way of obtaining them is small. Therefore, we
think that sound guidelines would forbid such an intervention. The
deontologist will justify such guidelines on the basis of the rights of
the child, and claim that these rights themselves require no further
justification. The utilitarian will agree that the child should be
accorded these rights, but justify the according of them, and the
actual guidelines, by appeal to the evil consequences that will
ensue if the rights are not safeguarded: loss of confidence in the
medical profession being only one of these.

The different approaches of deontologists and utilitarians to
problems such as we face can be further illustrated by a more
extreme, but hypothetical, example which is unlikely actually to
confront an ethics committee, but is typical of the imaginary cases
adduced by deontologists in their arguments with utilitarians. The
utilitarians, if they know the ropes, will protest that such unlikely
examples are a bad guide to practice in more usual cases ('hard
cases make bad law'). We have not found any actual examples in
which a utilitarian of the sort we are considering would be com-
mitted to approving flagrant violations of commonly accepted
human rights. In all the actual cases of high risk known to us, either
the research was of insufficient value to be justified by a risk/benefit
analysis, or there were other less dangerous ways of completing the
research. Since our task is to find guidelines for use in actual cases
not imaginary ones, the latter are irrelevant to our practical
problem.

However, waiving this objection by utilitarians, suppose that a
brain physiologist, on the basis of highly supportive animal
experiments, made a scientifically sound proposal for direct
experiments on the brains of psychotic infants using implanted
microelectrodes, direct brain biopsy and other invasive but only
moderately life-threatening methods; and suppose that there was
not much doubt, on the evidence, that such experiments would be
quite likely to afford a basis for important advances in medical
understanding of the biophysical basis of these disorders and thus
in their treatment and prevention. Should the rule against harming

the individual then be obeyed, or should it be ignored in favour of the course of action judged to give the greatest expectation of utility; namely, allowing the experiment? Should the children's parents be even *asked* for consent to such procedures?

A utilitarian of the sophisticated sort we are considering might seek to avoid this commitment. He might say that if ethics committees are to act for the best, they ought to form for themselves strict guidelines and stick to them. It is, he might say, very unlikely that any set of guidelines that was acceptable even from a purely utilitarian point of view would permit such experiments. For if it were known that ethics committees permitted this sort of thing, there would be widespread public revulsion prejudicing not merely medical research but the entire standing of the medical profession, to the great detriment of health care. People would cease to trust their doctors.

It would be of no use to the deontologist to suggest that the experiments might be kept secret; for this is not the sort of thing that can be concealed for long, and the research would be of little value unless published. Nor would it do for him to suggest that in a different sort of society (Nazi Germany, for example) arrangements could be made to carry out such experiments without interference from the public; for the utilitarian has good grounds for condemning such regimes in general, as likely to do much more harm than good to their subjects and the world. The deontologist might, however, claim that the utilitarian's argument has only succeeded on the basis of an assumption that the public's sentiments are unalterable; they are disposed to be outraged by such practices, and the outrage would rebound on the entire system of health care; so the practices should be forbidden. But what if the public itself could be converted to utilitarianism? Could not public and researchers then approve such experiments and worse?

To this the utilitarian might reply that this would not be 'a conversion to utilitarianism', because such a change in attitudes would be itself undesirable from the utilitarian point of view. If the public and doctors could approve such procedures, it would be a sign that there was something radically wrong with their attitudes – something that would lead to much greater harm than good in society as a whole. One could not, he might say, treat children (any children) as disposable in this way without entirely altering one's attitude to children in general and even to adults as well. One would be on a slippery slope which might really lead to support for a regime like that of the Nazis. The data for moral thinking include facts about what attitudes are humanly combinable; if *in practice* to let one principle go will lead to the sacrifice of a whole lot more, that is a reason for stopping earlier rather than later. Precisely where one should stop can be a matter for debate; but the utilitarian is allowed by his theory to have as strong views about this as anybody else, provided that the facts of our actual situation support them. The 'slippery slope' argument has, no doubt, often been abused, because not all slopes are *in practice* slippery (there are firm resting-places on many of them); but this one clearly is.

It is only apparently paradoxical for our sophicated utilitarian to say that ethics committees should not, in considering individual cases, always think in terms of utilities, or that the public ought not to be encouraged to do likewise. It will be remembered that the kind of utilitarian that we are considering thinks morally at two levels. It is perfectly self-consistent for him to recognize the utilitarian basis of all thinking, but to recognize also that this itself requires him, when considering practical proposals, to be guided by firm principles (of the same sort as the deontologist has adopted for his own kinds of reason), because that is the most likely way on the whole of acting for the best.

However, for the deontologist who is unconvinced by such argument and who finds reliance upon an overriding appeal to welfare maximization abhorrent – there are many, including members of the working group – the same working principles are derivable from other moral premises. Thus, those who hold as morally fundamental the Kantian principle that people should not be treated merely as means but always also as ends, and interpret this principle, unlike utilitarians, as ruling out such an appeal, will in practice – if they are not absolutists – find themselves upholding the same working rules as the utilitarian who supports such working rules on the grounds that they maximize welfare.

It is beyond the scope of this enquiry to pursue further this philosophical dispute. We have perhaps said enough to show that thoughtful utilitarians and deontologists, who have taken good cognizance of the relevant facts, may well agree in practice, as we have, on the guidelines to be adopted by ethics committees, and agree also in insisting that they should be firmly adhered to. That, at any rate, is the hope that has governed our detailed discussion of the issues. The two schools of thought will differ about the reasons to be given for these guidelines, or about the necessity for giving reasons at all; but into these further differences it is for our purposes unnecessary to enter.

References

1. Ross, W. D. *The right and the good,* p.41, Oxford University Press, Oxford (1930).
2. Prichard, H. A. Does moral philosophy rest on a mistake? *Mind* **XXI,** 21–37 (1912), reprinted in H. A. Prichard, *Moral obligation.* Oxford University Press (1949).
3. Warnock, G. J. *The object of morality,* pp.87 and 163. Methuen, London (1971).
4. Griffin, J. P. Modern Utilitarianism. *Revue internationale de philosophie, Bruxelles* **147,** 331–75 (1983).
5. Dworkin, R. M. *Taking rights seriously,* p.xv. Harvard University Press, Boston (1977).

5

Risks and benefits in
research on children

'Certain, 'tis certain; very sure, very sure: death, as the Psalmist saith, is certain to all; all shall die.'

Shakespeare allowed Justice Shallow in his senile chatter to recognize the one certain element of a human life: that it will end in death. All else in life, even the manner of death – whether it be peacefully in bed, as the result of crossing a road, or as the result of being a subject of clinical research – is uncertain. It is possible, however, to assess the statistical probability of a particular person dying in a particular way, though not necessarily very accurately. Such a calculation is an example of risk assessment.

Risk assessment is an activity in which everyone is daily involved: risks are a fact of life. Even the simplest activities have a measure of risk, though it may be very small. Drinking a glass of water in the United Kingdom is likely to carry only a very small risk of morbidity to most people; it is conceivable of course that it might 'go down the wrong way' and predispose to a chest infection or even cause drowning. The cumulative risk of morbidity could be greater if the water had passed through lead pipes. But if the drinker lived in rural Bangladesh, then the risk of mortality or morbidity would be several orders of magnitude greater – because of the possibility of contracting cholera or other water-borne infections. This is an example of an environmental risk, similar to those mentioned in Chapter 3 amongst the findings of the Black Report; environmental risks include risks to which people are exposed by virtue of the social class or the place in which they live. In many parts of Bangladesh inhabitants who are already disadvantaged are put at further risk because they cannot afford to buy clean water.

It was observed in the Introduction that the British Paediatric

Association's 'Guidelines to aid ethical committees considering research involving children'[1] depend in large part on the assessment of the risk/benefit ratio for any research activity on children. Similarly, the previous chapter has indicated that such risk/benefit analysis underlies both the utilitarian approach to making moral decisions and most of the compromise approaches that try to take account of a purely deontological viewpoint. It is, therefore, of considerable importance in a study of the ethics of clinical research investigations on children to examine the ways in which risk/benefit analyses are carried out, the limitations on their accuracy, and their value in making decisions.

Before discussing the nature of risk/benefit analysis and its possible value in assessing proposals for research on children, it would be wise to define some of the terms that will be used. The following definitions are those provided in a Royal Society report *Risk assessment*:[2]

(a) *Risk* is 'the probability that a particular *adverse event* occurs during a stated period of time or results from a particular challenge.'
(b) 'An *adverse event* is an occurrence that produces *harm*.'
(c) A *hazard* is 'the situation that in particular circumstances could lead to *harm*.'
(d) '*Harm* is the loss to a human being (or to a human population) consequent on *damage*.'
(e) '*Damage* is the loss of inherent quality suffered by an entity (physical or biological).'

The process of risk assessment can also be divided into three sections:

(i) risk identification, i.e. a qualitative description;
(ii) risk estimation, i.e. a quantitative description;
(iii) risk evaluation.[3] Risk evaluation is primarily a qualitative process in which the perceptions of a risk by those involved in any way with that risk are combined with the results of risk identification and estimation to produce a decision either to accept or reduce the risk. It will become apparent that such decisions do not rest purely on the numerical value assigned to a risk, but are determined in large part by a person's perception of the risk.

The Royal Society report defines benefit also:

'*Benefit* is the gain to a human population. Expected benefit incorporates an estimate of the probability of achieving the gain.'[2]

The concepts and measures defined above allow one to construct a framework within which one may attempt to carry out risk/benefit analyses with considerably greater rigour than most researchers have used heretofore. The BPA Guidelines, for instance, provided for the first time a number of examples of risk/benefit analysis in the assessment of proposals for research on children.[1] Yet the definitions of different degrees of risk were so vague that it was inevitable that some distinctly curious results were obtained, such as that referred to in the Introduction, when it was suggested that renal biopsy might be permissible in non-therapeutic research. It will be suggested in this chapter that much greater precision in risk/benefit analysis is already possible, but that there are at present inadequate data available to produce such precision in every assessment of research on children.

Risk identification

Risk assessment begins with risk identification, i.e. identification of situations in which adverse events, defined previously as hazards, may occur, and of the harms which may result from those adverse events. In research on children, each project will produce a number of different possible hazards for the subject children, even if the probability of harm resulting from them is extremely small. Parents and research ethics committees, in deciding to allow the participation of children in a research project, want to know the overall risk to which they expose the children as a result of that decision. Unless the project involves only a single intervention, it will be necessary to identify the hazards of each intervention and add together the risks arising. Most of the risks of medical procedures discussed later in this chapter are those which arise from a single intervention; it should be noted that the risks of everyday life with which they are compared are usually related to travelling a certain number of miles or carrying out an activity for a certain number of hours.

An opportunity to illustrate risk identification is provided by the example of percutaneous liver biopsy: there have been several recent reports[4-6] of research projects during which this procedure was performed on children. The biopsy itself may produce a number of hazards, amongst which are intraperitoneal bleeding, pneumothorax, biliary peritonitis, bacteraemia, and death.[7] Before performing any liver biopsy, however, it is mandatory to perform clotting studies on the individual child's blood. In the process of hazard identification for liver biopsy one should therefore include also the hazards of obtaining a blood sample. These are extremely numerous including haemorrhage, thrombophlebitis, venous thrombosis, infections such as cellulitis, septicaemia, septic arthritis or osteomyelitis, bruising, pain at the sample site, fainting and occasionally even cardiac arrest, and damage to the child from restraint used during the procedure.[8-10]

The above lists concentrate on the physical hazards that are relatively straightforward to identify. They do not include emotional or psychological hazards, nor hazards to other members of the child's family, which may be less obvious. A child may suffer varying degrees of emotional distress, either as a result of pain or discomfort felt during the research procedure, or as a result of being in unfamiliar surroundings. Parents may also become distressed, and feel guilt in particular, when they observe in practice what they have allowed to be done to their children. There is some evidence that participation in a research project may also uncover tensions within a family with which the family had previously coped.[11] These various forms of possible emotional distress represent hazards that may need to be included in the risk/benefit analysis of a particular project.

The third category of hazards that must be considered during risk identification is those to which a subject or his family would not have been exposed, had it not been for his participation in the research project, but which do not arise from the particular research procedure used. One might include in this category the hazard of merely being in a hospital physically;[12] two of the harms to which this may lead are hospital-acquired infection, and accidents caused by unfamiliar surroundings. If in addition parents have, for instance, to drive their child to hospital for a visit that would not otherwise have been necessary, then one must include amongst the identified risks the hazard of driving however many miles it may be. It will be evident, however, from the figures given later in this chapter for the risks of various modes of travel that there will only be occasional instances when the distance travelled to hospital will be great enough to constitute a risk that might not be ignored.

Risk estimation

The next part of risk assessment to be considered is risk estimation, which in itself involves two separate elements: first, a probability determination which can in principle be an objective measure, and second, an estimate of the harm of any adverse event that will usually be more subjective. In the previous example of risk identification, various possible adverse events following the collection of a blood specimen were noted. It should be possible to measure the probability of any given adverse event occurring, whether in research or routine clinical practice, even though the confidence limits of the probability may be quite wide. No such measurement appears ever to have been undertaken, however, for adverse events consequent on the collection of blood specimens, although figures are available for other hazards.

The second element in risk estimation consists in the determination of the relative magnitude, or disutility, of each harm that might occur. A life-threatening harm such as septicaemia obviously carries a far greater disutility than transient bruising or tenderness at the site of the venepuncture. How then might one develop a scale of disutility? One possible solution would be to try to translate all possible harms into financial values. An illustration of an attempt to do this is provided by the Department of Transport's estimates of the costs to society of road accidents. The cost elements include loss of output, ambulance and hospital costs, and a notional figure for pain, grief, and suffering. The 1981 estimates [13] range from £130 for a slight casualty to £132 700 for a fatality. Such estimates are very limited and could only provide a small part of a scale of disutility that would in any case be directed more to the interests of society than the interests of individuals. Further parts of the scale might be derived from the sums awarded by the courts as damages for particular harms. But the scale would remain incomplete: life and health cannot be bought, and so any financial valuation must in the end be inadequate.

Other attempts have been made to construct scales of the disutility of various harms by philosophers, psychologists, and health economists, since there are various obvious uses to which a generally accepted gradation of harm or disability might be put. Philosophers have tended to base their assessments of utility and disutility on the idea of preference satisfaction. Thus, harm would be assessed according to the strength of preference of the person affected that the harm should not happen. Rowe suggested a 'Hierarchy of risk consequences' based on the conceptual hierarchy of human needs suggested by Maslow, an American humanistic psychologist.[3] The essence of the hierarchy is the supposition that as basic needs, such as the avoidance of premature death, are satisfied so other, higher, needs such as finding food or shelter, protecting one's rights or property, achieving love and a sense of belonging, successively take the place of more basic needs as motives for human action. If a hazard threatens the fulfilment of a need, then the more basic the need, the greater the potential harm.

Many of the health indicators developed by economists do not seem to offer any direct help in the estimation of research risks. A scale of valuations of thirty different states of illness developed by Rosser, a psychiatrist, however, seems to offer a glimmer of hope that scales could be developed that would allow direct comparison of different harms that might arise as the result of research on children.[14] She asked seventy adults to compare eight different states of disability with four different states of distress superimposed on each. From the results she was able to develop a table (Table 5.5, see p. 109) showing the relative degree of undesirability of each state as perceived by her seventy respondents. The table is by no means complete and refers only to adults: it may well be that states of disability and distress of children might be perceived differently. It does, however, offer the possibility of using the same scale to measure both the magnitude of possible harms in a research project and the magnitude of possible benefits. Examples of how this might be done are given later in the chapter.

One is left with the conclusion that there is as yet no quantifiable scale of values that is comprehensive enough to allow one directly to compare, for instance, pneumothorax after a liver biopsy with the stress and anxiety caused to the child by the performance of that liver biopsy. Inevitably, a value judgement will have to be made, and can only be made by the subject himself, or his parents or guardian. It is important to note that this value judgement should only be of the relative magnitude of a harm: it is not a value judgement of the entire risk. All too often in medical activities risks are assessed intuitively, and, as in the BPA Guidelines, the probability of an adverse event occurring is not distinguished and measured separately from the disutility of the harm caused.

Risk evaluation

The third part of risk assessment that falls to be considered is risk evaluation, the process of combining the results of risk identification and estimation with the perceptions of those involved in order to come to a decision about a risk. A report of the Council for Science and Society[15] stresses the need for assessment to be undertaken by the person exposed: 'The judgement of "acceptability" of a risk involves a consideration of its perceived costs and benefits in the light of feasible alternatives, *by the person exposed to it*' (their emphasis). This is an essential part of risk assessment because there is an enormous variety in the ways in which risks are perceived. The high risks of activities such as riding a motorcycle are readily accepted by the participants, while risks that are several orders of magnitude smaller, such as the release of radioactive matter from nuclear power stations, may not be widely accepted. This comparison illustrates an important distinction: voluntary risks are more readily accepted than involuntary ones. Indeed, part of the value of participating in high-risk sports such as mountaineering or hang-gliding may be considered by the participants to be the need to learn how to face possible death or injury. The example of the risk of release of radioactive matter from a nuclear power station also illustrates another important point about risk perception: the same risk may be perceived, and therefore evaluated, in very different ways by different people. Those who work in nuclear power stations and who might be expected to understand the risks are in general ready to accept them, while members of the public who may lack a precise understanding of the nature and magnitude of the risks are most likely to reject them. The greatest differences in perception of a risk often seem to arise between those who are supposed to know about it and those who do not. These differences may be related not only to differing valuations of a particular harm, but also to the difficulties inherent in making sense of mathematical probabilities.

Various examples may be given of the variations in the evaluation of the risk of death. Ashby[16] looks at the example of deaths in road and aircraft accidents in the United States. About 150 people are killed on the roads each day, but such carnage has no impact on the public. Yet, when 350 people died in an air crash, a shock wave went round the country, and indeed the world, with all sorts of enquiries being set up. Card and Mooney[17] looked at the amount of money that society was willing to pay in order to prevent a death from various possible causes. The results showed an enormous variation, from £1000 to prevent a child being poisoned, by introducing child-resistant medicine containers, through the cost of £100 000 to prevent death when a tractor rolls over by the provision of a rigid cab, to £20 000 000 by changing the building regulations after the partial collapse of a block of flats called Ronan Point in the East End of London. The basis of such calculations may be illustrated by the agricultural tractor example. Approximately forty fatal accidents used to occur each year, either to tractor drivers, or often to children riding on the back of a tractor, when the tractor accidentally rolled over. It was decided by Parliament that such accidents were not acceptable, and legislation was passed requiring all new tractors to be fitted with a rigid cab. The cost of the rigid cabs added £4 000 000 each year to the price of tractors bought in this country, a cost of £100 000 for each of the lives that might be saved. Since tractor drivers and passengers are still sometimes killed in roll-over accidents, the true cost of each life saved is even higher.

The Royal Society definition given earlier stated that risk is 'the probability that a particular adverse event occurs during a stated period of time, or results from a particular challenge.' The most frequently measured 'adverse event' is death, since the most complete records are available through death certificates and other sources. The information that would be most useful in assessing proposals for research on children – measures of the incidence of injuries as a result of various research procedures – is often not available. The available information about the risk of death in various activities is nevertheless of considerable value in trying to decide what levels of voluntary and involuntary risks are acceptable in our society. Such decisions are often extremely difficult and are reminiscent of a story, told by Kletz, 'about a civil servant who spent a holiday working on a farm. One day he was asked to sort a pile of potatoes into large ones and small ones. By the end of the day he had sorted 10 and was on the edge of a nervous breakdown – he found the decisions difficult to make because he had no criterion for deciding which potatoes were large and which were small.'[18]

Risks of everyday life

Table 5.1   Annual UK occupational fatality risks[19]
(1974–8 except as stated)

	Risk per million
Manufacture of clothing and footwear	4
Manufacture of vehicles	15
Manufacture of timber, furniture, etc.	40
Chemical and allied industries	85
Shipbuilding and marine engineering	100
Agriculture (employees)	100
Construction industries	150
Railway staff	180
Coal miners	210
Quarrying	300
Offshore oil and gas workers (1967–76)	1600
Deep sea fishing (accidents at sea only, 1959–68)	2800

Table 5.1 shows the risk of accidental death to which workers in various occupations are exposed for each year that they work. The figure of four per million for workers in the manufacture of clothing and footwear means that of each million workers in that industry four per annum are likely to have a fatal accident at work. In this chapter, risks will be described either as being X per million, or, when the numbers might be unwieldy, as Y per thousand. It is possible to represent these mathematically as $X \times 10^{-6}$ and $Y \times 10^{-3}$, and to use other powers of the base 10 also, but readers may find risks easier to compare when they are all represented as being either per million or per thousand. As one looks down Table 5.1, the numerical values of the risks become greater: the risk of a fatal accident during deep-sea fishing is 2800 per million, a risk that is 700 times greater than the risk of a fatal accident during the manufacture of clothing and footwear. Thus, it can be seen that in practice people are willing to accept a large range in the magnitude of the risks to which they are exposed by virtue of their work. (The extent to which such risks are environmental risks – i.e. determined by geography and the lack of alternative employment – is too complex a question to be considered here, but does suggest a constraint on the voluntariness of employment in certain fields.) The risk figures given in Table 5.1 apply only to fatal accidents,

however; workers in some industries have been exposed to much greater risks of developing cancer by virtue of exposure to various chemicals. Uranium mining, for instance, used to present a risk of 1500 deaths/million/year from lung cancer, in addition to the risk of a fatal accident: the latter varies in mining from country to country, but lies in the range of 200 to 1000 million/year;[20] the risk of lung cancer is now thought to be substantially lower.

Table 5.2 Risk of fatality to passengers, per 100 miles travelled, UK[19] (1972–6)

	Risk per million
By rail (train accidents)	0.07
In public service vehicles	0.19
By UK airlines (scheduled services)	0.22
By car or taxi	1.1
By pedal cycle	14
By motorbicycle, etc. ('2-wheeled motor vehicles')	
driver	26
passenger	57

Table 5.2 shows the risk of death incurred by travelling 100 miles by various means of transport. Once again a substantial difference may be seen between degrees of risk voluntarily accepted by members of the general public: a pillion passenger on a motorcycle is about 800 times more likely to die than a rail passenger.

Table 5.3 shows the risk of death in various sports that could probably be recognized as high-risk sports even without the confirmation of these figures. One sport that, perhaps surprisingly, carries a considerably lower risk of fatality is full-bore target rifle shooting. In the United Kingdom there have been no fatalities in the last 30 years, over which period the risk of being hit by a bullet is 7 per million per participant year. This sport does, however, illustrate the morbidity that sportsmen may accept as a result of their sport. A recent survey[21] showed that 68 per cent of those who had been shooting for 25 years or more had a hearing loss averaging more than 50 decibels between 3000 and 6000 Hz, which would cause significant disability both at work and socially. Many other sports also produce significant morbidity, which may perhaps be illustrated best by the recent development of the new speciality of sports medicine.

Table 5.3   Risk of death in sporting activities[19]

	Risk per million
Per participant year	
Cave exploration (US, 1970–78)	50
Scuba diving (UK, sub-aqua club members 1970–80)	200
Glider flying (US, 1970–80)	400
Power boat racing (US, 1970–78)	800
Hang gliding (UK, Hang Gliding Assocn, 1977–79)	1500
Sport parachuting (US, 1978)	2000
Per participant hour	
Amateur boxing (UK, 1946–62)	0.5
Skiing (US, 1967–68, France 1974–76) about	1
Canoeing (UK, 1960–62)	10
Mountaineering (US, 1951–60)	30
Rock climbing (UK, 1961)	40

Table 5.4   One in a million risk of death from the following

Three-quarters of a cigarette
50 miles by car
250 miles by air
1½ min rock climbing
6 min canoeing
20 min being a man aged 60
1 day being a boy aged 12
1 or 2 weeks' typical factory work

Table 5.4 draws together some of the activities that cause a risk of death of one per million. Were one to multiply all the hazards by a factor of 10, so that the risk became 10 per million, it is likely that all would remain equally acceptable to the great majority of members of the public. Multiplying by a factor of 100, however, might push some of the risks close to the limits of acceptability. 5000 miles is, in fact, very close to the average distance travelled by car by each member of the population of the United Kingdom every year,[22] and is presumably therefore generally acceptable. Flying 25 000 miles, on the other hand, might give some people pause for thought: as Knox points out, insurance companies are able to sell additional insurance against such a risk to a reasonable number of air passengers.[23] A cigarette smoker who smoked 20 cigarettes per day would have to use a much larger multiplying factor – approximately 10 000 – to calculate his annual risk of death, which would be about 10 000 per million, or 10 per thousand. Such a risk is greater than the annual risk of death from all other causes up to the ages of 55 for a male, or 65 for a female.[22] Not only smokers, however, should remember the American bumper sticker: 'Life is hazardous to your health'.

The figures given in the tables show the magnitude of risks that are voluntarily accepted, and also the wide range in the risks of daily life for different members of the population. It is readily evident that a definition, such as that in the BPA Guidelines, of negligible risk as 'risk less than that run in everyday life' is effectively meaningless. The only alternative would be to accept the idea that negligible risk is relative to the risk to which a child is already exposed: the higher the risk to which a child is already exposed, the higher the level of risk in a research procedure on that child which can be neglected. Such an idea is intolerable. One cannot draw any conclusion as to which risks are neglected when the figures given range from 680 per thousand for hearing loss in rifle shooters, to something between 10 and 100 per million for death in airline passengers on a typical long-haul flight, to less than 0.1 per million for release of radioactive matter from nuclear power stations.[18] Knox suggests that 'the best indications of the lower limits of non-neglected risks probably come from medical sources'.[23] This is fortunate since it would perhaps be reasonable to suggest that risk/benefit ratios in medical research or in medical practice that were of the same order of magnitude might in general be equally acceptable.

Negligible risks in medicine

The risks of immunization provide useful information, the more so since the aim of immunization is to protect against a potential illness, rather than to treat an actual illness, and is therefore rather closer to medical research in risk/benefit implications than most of medical practice. Between 1951 and 1970 15.5 million smallpox vaccinations were carried out, resulting in 77 deaths and 574 other severe complications, giving risks of 5 per million for death, and 37 per million for severe complications.[24] These risks were accepted even when smallpox had become an extremely rare disease in this country, so that the prospect of benefit to an infant was extremely small. More recently, the overall fatality risk for the eight most common immunizations has been of the order of one per million.[25] The risk of morbidity from whooping-cough immunization has, however, attracted much public attention. Retrospective analysis suggested that the risk of permanent brain damage might be 40 per million, i.e. a similar risk to that previously accepted for severe complications of smallpox vaccination.[26] The publicity given to the possibility of brain damage, however, ensured that the proportion of infants immunized against whooping-cough dropped from 78 per cent in 1973 to 32 per cent in 1978. Prospective analysis now suggests that the risk of brain damage is closer to 10 per million for each infant receiving a course of three injections, and uptake of whooping-cough immunization has now crept up to about 55 per cent. It is tempting to suggest that a risk of 10 per million of major morbidity is therefore ignored by about one-half of parents, but there are many other influences on their decisions.

A similar conclusion can be drawn from the 'Swine Flu Affair' in 1976 in the United States. A young army recruit was found to have died in February 1976 of an influenza virus, known as swine flu, that was very similar to the virus that had caused the 1918–19 influenza pandemic.[27] As a result it was decided to undertake a massive immunization programme of the whole population of the United States the following autumn. Six weeks after the start of the immunization programme reports started of an increase in the incidence of Guillain–Barré syndrome, an uncommon neurological condition usually producing transient paralysis, but occasionally ending in permanent paralysis or death. After 45 million doses of the swine-flu vaccine had been given, 427 cases of Guillain–Barré syndrome were recognized in people who had received the vaccine, i.e. a risk of approximately 10 per million. This was sufficient for the immunization programme to be suspended by President Carter.

A rather different medical example is that of taking the contraceptive pill. Knox,[23] using figures obtained at a time when 'first-generation' contraceptive pills, with a relatively high dose of oestrogen, were in use, suggests a risk of death of 500 per million for a reproductive lifetime of continuous pill-taking. This risk was thought by many women to be too high, and there was considerable public approval of the Committee on Safety of

Medicines' decision to limit the allowable amount of oestrogen in the contraceptive pill to a low dose.

The World Health Organization and the International Commission on Radiological Protection have examined the risks of various doses of radiation, whether from radiological examination or the use of radionuclides in order to 'scan' particular organs. The majority of both sorts of investigation delivers a radiation dose of less than 5 millisieverts.[28] The risks of such a dose (5 mSv) to children would be about 100 per million for a substantial genetic abnormality in the descendants of the irradiated individual, and about 60 per million for a fatal subsequent malignancy in the exposed child.[25] The latter risk is very similar to the risk of a fatal malignancy developing in a child born after a single antenatal X-ray of his mother's abdomen – 61 per million in the 1960s Oxford Survey.[29] Such a risk has often been accepted by obstetricians but only after due consideration and certainly not routinely; the increased availability of ultrasound has now greatly reduced the need for such examinations.

The risks of taking medicaments have been examined by Girdwood, using data received by the Committee on Safety of Medicines.[30] He was able to produce a rough guide to the dangers of various medicines by dividing the number of deaths reported to the CSM as being caused by a particular drug during a three-year period by the number of prescriptions for the drug in the same period. It is necessarily only a rough guide, since it is impossible to know what proportion of adverse reactions to drugs are actually reported to the CSM; moreover, the counting of general practitioners' prescriptions alone excludes any information about the use of the drugs in hospital practice. The figures that he obtained showed that 22 drugs produced a risk of death per prescription greater than 1 per million, 6 drugs produced a risk greater than 10 per million, and 1 drug used in the treatment of rheumatoid arthritis produced a risk of 160 per million. Experience recently with a different anti-arthritic drug, benoxaprofen, suggests that the latter risk of death is now unacceptable, and throws some doubt on the risk of 10 per million being acceptable.

The evidence of these medical examples suggests that in medical practice a risk of death of one per million is indeed neglected by both doctors and the general public. Risks of the order of 10 per million, however, whether of death or of severe non-fatal consequences, are not in general ignored by non-medical people, although they may be neglected by doctors. It appears that the borderline of negligibility for doctors probably lies at about 50 per million, although larger risks are effectively ignored when the patient's condition already puts him at a high risk of death.

Risks of medical procedures

1. Blood sampling

Having reached this tentative conclusion about what risks are in practice neglected, it is necessary to outline what is known of the risks of various adverse events occurring during clinical research on children, even though it may not be possible to quantify the harm that arises from such adverse events. Probably the commonest procedure undertaken in clinical research is the obtaining of a specimen of venous blood. There are occasional anecdotal reports giving accounts of adverse events, such as those listed earlier, that may occur; although McKay commented in 1966[8] that there was inadequate statistical data on adverse events, no attempt seems to have been made since to gather such information for venepuncture. It may be that there is reluctance to do so, particularly in the United States, for medico-legal reasons. The Report of the Secretary's Commission on Medical Malpractice states that: 'There appears to be reluctance on the part of some physicians to publish in medical journals case reports, describing in detail noted adverse effects of diagnostic and therapeutic procedures, because of the fear that the material will be used as evidence in a lawsuit.'[31]

Two recent reports provide a little information about the psychological effects on young children of a non-therapeutic venepuncture. In both cases the reason for obtaining blood specimens was to survey blood lead levels. In the first study,[32] Rodin wanted to assess the effect on a child's anxiety level during venepuncture of using games in preparing the child. The children, aged 4 to 7 years, spent a few minutes in a waiting room, either playing with a specially prepared medical game showing what was about to happen to them, or playing with ordinary commercially produced games, or having no play materials. Those using the special game had higher levels of observed anxiety in the waiting room, which diminished during venepuncture; the other two groups showed an increase in anxiety so that, on average, unprepared children were not co-operative, were hesitant, not wanting to talk, looking tense, and often crying. The prepared children, whose parents had also warned them what was to happen, were on average co-operative, responsive, and only occasionally showing signs of tension. Interestingly, in a study sponsored by the National Association for the Welfare of Children in Hospital, the parents appear only to have been asked for consent to the venepuncture on their children, and not for consent to their children's participation in the anxiety study. The other recent study, from the Institute of Child Health,[33] reports a questionnaire survey undertaken 18 months after a group of 92 children had provided blood samples for a different survey of blood lead levels, with parental consent. The questionnaires were addressed to the parents and 77 were returned. Ninety-two per cent of parents said that their children had not been upset at all by the venepuncture, while 8 per cent said that their children had been mildly upset, but for no longer than one day. Seven per cent of the children had complained of a sore arm, 8 per cent had had some bruising and 85 per cent had no physical after-effects. Forty per cent of the parents thought that the experience had made their children slightly or definitely more confident when attending a doctor or dentist subsequently. These results need to be viewed in the light of their having been obtained a considerable time after the event.

While little is known of the risks of entering veins, there have been some reports of the adverse effects of peripheral arterial puncture: they relate, however, to events in adults, and may not therefore be directly comparable to possible adverse events in children. Mortensen reported in 1967 on 3193 arterial entries performed between 1961 and 1966 either by needle puncture, by cannulation, or by incision.[34] In this series there were, as a result of arterial entry, 4 deaths, 2 limb amputations, 4 residual deficits as a result of strokes, 56 other major complications, and 321 minor complications, such as persistent severe pain, local swelling, or temporary loss of the distal pulse. These figures give a risk of fatality of 1.3 per thousand, a risk of residual serious damage of 2 per thousand, an overall risk of major complication of 22 per thousand, and a risk of minor complications of 100 per thousand; however, such risk estimates bear little or no relation to present practice.

The techniques of arterial puncture have become much safer since 1967 so that death, in particular, is now a rare outcome. A report in 1979 from a London hospital[35] gave the results of 839 arterial punctures performed at 580 sites in 282 patients, either under local anaesthesia or during general anaesthesia. When each puncture site was examined between one and three days after the procedure, nine were found to have bruising greater than 2 centi-metres in diameter and one site was still tender enough for the patient to complain spontaneously of pain. Another patient was found to have developed an aneurysm at the puncture site. The risk of significant complications was therefore about 19 per thousand puncture sites. Some degree of pain, tenderness, bruis-ing or diminution of the distal pulse was present one to three days later at a further 226 of the puncture sites, giving a risk of minor complications of 390 per thousand sites. It should be noted that, in practice, arterial punctures are often performed without local ana-esthesia, when there will invariably be some pain.

2. Cardiothoracic procedures

Over the last twenty-five years the investigation of congenital and other forms of heart disease has been greatly assisted by two deve-lopments: the use of ultrasound, in the technique known as echo-cardiography, and cardiac catheterization. In the latter procedure a flexible tube, a catheter, is passed through a large vein or artery in the arm or groin, or in neonates the umbilicus, and advanced into the heart. Direct measurements may be made of the blood pressure in the various chambers of the heart or in the great vessels; blood may be sampled from the same sites to measure its oxygen concentration; and radio-opaque dye may be injected dir-ectly into various parts of the heart while X-rays or an X-ray video film are made. The procedure may also be used for therapy, either by creating a communication between two heart chambers that do not normally communicate in order to relieve some other abnor-mality, or, in adults, by enlarging the bore of coronary arteries that are narrowed or blocked.

The largest review of the complications of this procedure is that of Rudolph published in 1968.[36] He reviewed the outcome of the procedure in 4208 infants and children, and recorded a long list of possible complications. These included hypotension (low blood-pressure), bradycardia (a slow pulse), respiratory arrest, cyanotic episodes, obstruction of either a coronary artery or one of the out-lets of the heart, cardiac failure, perforation of the heart or great vessels directly or by injection of radio-opaque contrast medium, and infections. There were also the complications of entering an artery referred to earlier. Rudolph showed that the risk of a fatal outcome was much greater in the first two months of life than subsequently. It must be remembered, however, that infants of that age requiring cardiac catheterization are often seriously ill before the procedure, and that it takes little in some cases to tip the balance against survival. In the first week of life, Rudolph showed that the risk of death was 85 per thousand; for the first month of life, overall, it was 77 per thousand and in the second month it was 52 per thousand. For the remainder of the first year, the risk of death was 13 per thousand; from 1 year old to 15 years the risk of death was even lower – 2 per thousand. The risks of non-fatal complications showed a similar gradation: in the first two months, the risk was 81 per thousand, dropping to 34 per thousand for the remainder of the first year of life, and 15 per thousand in the 1 to 15 years age range.

The report [37] of a smaller series of infants the following year produced a similar result to one of Rudolph's. During a series of 100 cardiac catheterizations at the Johns Hopkins Hospital in infants aged under one month, there were 6 fatalities attributable to the procedure rather than to the disease of the infants. This gives a risk of death of 60 per thousand, while Rudolph's figure was 77 per thousand. A few years later, Miller reviewed the experience of the Brompton Hospital in London.[38] One hundred and eighteen infants had been submitted to cardiac catheterization during the first week of life: 2 had died as a result of the procedure and 12 had had complications as defined in the Rudolph survey. These results show a much lower risk of death – 17 per thousand compared to Rudolph's figure of 85 per thousand, but a somewhat higher risk of non-fatal complications – 102 per thousand.

A procedure that is occasionally carried out in children in order to help in the diagnosis of a mass seen on a chest X-ray is percutaneous needle biopsy of the lung. Allison and Hemingway[39] reported a series of 160 such biopsies in 149 patients aged between 9 and 86 years. The commonest complication was a pneumothorax which occurred after 38 biopsies; only twice, however, did this complication require any treatment. In 16 cases there were other problems, such as puncturing a blood vessel, haematoma formation, or haemoptysis (coughing up blood). None of these patients required any treatment. For this procedure, therefore, available evidence does not allow an estimate of the risk of death, but suggests that the risk of a major complication is 13 per thousand and that the risk of a minor complication is 325 per thousand. Since, however, the only evidence for most of the minor complications is found on X-rays taken after the procedure, patients would usually be unaware of them.

This report on needle biopsy of the lung also provides useful evidence that the more experience an investigator has in using a technique, the safer it is likely to be. The performance of one operator in the series of biopsies is given, showing that over a period of six years the incidence of pneumothorax dropped from 50 per cent to less than 20 per cent in patients biopsied by him.

3. Lumbar puncture

Lumbar puncture, the withdrawal of a specimen of cerebrospinal fluid from around the spinal cord by inserting a needle between two lumbar vertebrae, is commonly performed in children since it is an essential part of the diagnosis, amongst other conditions, of meningitis. A recent review in the *British Medical Journal* summed up the procedure thus: 'Lumbar puncture remains an essential neurological tool, with unpleasant if short-lived sequelae in many patients.'[40] The most common adverse effect is a quite severe headache, the possible origin of which is described in the same review as being attributable 'to leakage of cerebrospinal fluid through the hole in the dura, which leads to intracranial hypotension with traction on pain-sensitive nerve endings in the dura and intracranial vessels'. It appears to occur in at least one-quarter of all adults, but may be less common in children: the risk is likely to be of the order of 100 per thousand. There are a variety of less common adverse events in lumbar puncture that have mostly been described anecdotally, and that may cause serious harm. In certain conditions, and particularly when raised intracranial pressure has not been recognized, removal of cerebrospinal fluid by lumbar puncture may allow part of the brain stem to be extruded through the hole in the skull from which the spinal cord issues: this process is known as 'coning' and is often fatal. A small piece of skin may be introduced into the spinal canal and grow to form a dermoid tumour. It is not known how common either of these adverse events is.

One adverse event associated with lumbar puncture in children has however been quite well documented: the incidence of meningitis developing after lumbar puncture has been performed in children with bacteria in their blood. One paper in 1975[41] described four children, and reviewed a further seven cases from the literature, in which an initial lumbar puncture in an ill child had produced normal cerebrospinal fluid, but a subsequent lumbar puncture had shown meningitis. It was presumed that the performance of a lumbar puncture allowed small amounts of bacteraemic blood into the cerebrospinal fluid facilitating infection of the latter. More recently a group in Boston, USA, reported[42] on a group of 277 children only mildly or moderately ill when first seen; in fact, 90 per cent were sent home after initial assessment. All these children had a bacteraemia, and lumbar puncture was performed on 46 of them, in every case producing normal cerebrospinal fluid. Seven of the 46 who had lumbar puncture subsequently developed meningitis, while only 2 of the 231 children who did not have a lumbar puncture developed meningitis. This suggests that the risk of developing meningitis when a mildly or moderately ill child has a bacteraemia is 9 per thousand. But if a lumbar puncture is performed the risk becomes 152 per thousand: thus the additional risk of developing meningitis imposed on a bacteraemic child by the performance of a lumbar puncture is 143 per thousand. It should be noted that some clinicians would dispute the explanation given for the apparent association of a lumbar puncture performed during bacteraemia and the subsequent development of meningitis. They would suggest that good clinical judgement had allowed the physicians to select for lumbar puncture children in whom meningitis was developing, although the cerebrospinal fluid did not yet show any evidence of it. There is, however, experimental evidence from work on dogs[43] supporting the explanation that lumbar puncture allows small amounts of bacteraemic blood to enter and infect the cerebrospinal fluid.

One difficulty with lumbar puncture is that a considerable degree of skill is required in its performance: it is not automatically successful. One group in a neonatal intensive care unit in the US prospectively evaluated 289 attempts at lumbar puncture on infants in their unit:[44] 76 attempts were traumatic, in that there were more than 5000 red blood cells per cubic millimetre in the third tube of cerebrospinal fluid collected: 61 attempts were unsuccessful, in that no fluid was obtained. Thus, there was an overall failure rate of 47 per cent, which was shown not to be dependent on the sort of needle used. It is important, therefore, to note that on average two attempts will have to be made at every lumbar puncture on an infant, although one may hope that the success rate is greater in experienced hands than in a unit where many of the attempts were made by house staff.

The lack of information available about other adverse effects of lumbar puncture illustrates a more general point. The ignoring of adverse events can be viewed as a habit inculcated in medical training when much time may be spent on discussion of the complications of an illness, but little on the complications of diagnostic and therapeutic procedures other than drug treatment. A brief review of ten standard textbooks picked at random supports this point. The books included two on clinical methods, three on general medicine and five on paediatrics. In their accounts of lumbar puncture, one book mentioned headache as a possible consequence and another mentioned 'coning'. The other eight books mentioned no adverse effects, although most of them warned against the performance of lumbar puncture in the presence of raised intracranial pressure.

4. Gastroenterology

A Work Group of American gastroenterologists was formed at the request of the National Institute of Arthritis, Metabolism and Digestive Diseases in order to assemble information concerning the risks of procedures used in gastroenterology.[7] They admitted in many cases to finding the same problem as the present working group – that there is all too often inadequate documentation of adverse events either in research or in routine practice. They did, however, collect together much useful information, of which some items relevant to research on children are recorded below.

The passage of a nasogastric tube appeared to be a procedure that was almost free of serious complications: there is, of course, almost always some discomfort as it is passed. Anecdotal, but not quantitative, evidence was available to the American gastroenterologists about rare complications such as the development of peptic oesophagitis with long-term intubation, knotting of the tube in the stomach requiring removal by laparotomy, and perforation of the stomach. It was suggested that the risk of serious complications from nasogastric intubation was less than 10 per million. Peroral biopsy of the small intestine was not known to have produced any deaths or perforations of the intestine when performed with a Crosby capsule. The figures for the Crosby capsule gave an overall risk of bleeding of 2.4 per thousand, but for children only this was reduced to 1.4 per thousand. Rigid sigmoidoscopy as a procedure was thought to be very safe in children, but since it generally required the child to be sedated, a risk of fatality of 100 per million was suggested, approximating the risk of sedation. No data were available on the risks of fibreoptic gastrointestinal endoscopy, but enquiry had suggested that they were no greater than for adults. The risk of complications such as bleeding, perforation, or transmitted infections in adults was 1.32 per thousand.

Before the introduction of the Menghini needle for percutaneous liver biopsy, the risk of death from the procedure was 1700 per million.[45] Since its introduction, two surveys reported by the NIAMDD Work Group suggest a risk of death of 160 per million. The Liver Unit at King's College Hospital has more recently reported a similar risk of death of 200 per million.[46,47] Morbidity from the procedure is somewhat higher, the risk of a serious complication such as biliary peritonitis, pneumothorax or intraperitoneal bleeding being 4 per thousand. Knauer, however, has reported[48] a series of 1107 liver biopsies in which 6 major haemorrhages occurred giving a risk of 5.4 per thousand for that complication alone. The NIAMDD Work Group comments that 'it is unlikely that the risk of the procedure in children is inherently greater' than in adults, but also points out that the mortality and morbidity increase when the procedure is performed on a patient 'who is unable to co-operate by following instructions during the procedure'. One test of liver function used in research and clinical practice is the bromsulphthalein retention test: bromsulphthalein can produce a severe allergic reaction known as anaphylaxis. The risk of anaphylaxis in this test is about 6 per million, with a risk of death of 3 per million.[49]

5. General

The above information on quantifiable risks of various procedures performed on children represents all that could be found, other than anecdotal reports. There are obviously large gaps in this information, particularly where the risks of venepuncture are concerned. Another area in which information would be useful is in assessing the risks of sedation or anaesthesia, since sedation at least is required for the performance of many different procedures on children who would otherwise be unco-operative. It is known that the risk of death attributable to the general anaesthetic used in major surgical operations dropped from 600 per million in 1951 to 40 per million in 1973.[25] It would be reasonable to suppose that the risk is now of the order of 20 per million, but there is no obvious way of converting that to a figure for the risk of sedating children.

If one peruses paediatric journals, it is evident that trials of new drugs appear to be less frequent in children than in adults. It will not surprise the reader to know that no figures are available for the risks of such trials. Indeed, the only figures that do seem to be available for drug trials are those of Zarafonetis.[50] This study evaluated the incidence of adverse events in Phase I drug trials – i.e. trials of drugs before they have been licensed for use by the general public – carried out on inmates of the State Prison of Southern Michigan, the largest prison in the United States with over 5000 prisoners: 29 162 participants had been involved in 805 trials during a 12-year period. One subject taking a placebo died of a stroke; another had residual disability arising from septic arthritis of the hip following an injection of a corticosteroid. Otherwise, there was complete recovery from 58 adverse drug reactions and 4 other medical complications. It is impossible to be certain what role the placebo played in the one death, and therefore no figure can be calculated from these data for the risk of death from participating in a drug trial; the risk of serious harm could be calculated as 30 per million, but the confidence limits of such a calculation would be extremely wide. The risk of a significant medical complication would be approximately 2 per thousand; since a total of 614 534 subject days accumulated over that period, the risk of a significant medical complication could also be expressed as 100 per million for each day of a subject's exposure.

One other study provides some information averaged over a large number of research projects.[51] This was undertaken for the Department of Health, Education and Welfare in the United States when the Secretary of the Department wished to know the size of the problem before deciding whether to compensate research subjects who suffered injury. The figures for injuries in therapeutic research are probably of little value to this present study since most occurred during trials of chemotherapy for various cancers. There were, however, 93 399 subjects of non-therapeutic research who had suffered a total of 711 injuries, of which 673 were trivial, 37 were temporarily disabling, and 1 was permanently disabling; there had been no deaths. Trivial injuries included discomfort after aspiration of a joint, scars after punch biopsy of the skin, haematomata after venepuncture, colds induced for study purposes, corneal abrasions, reactions to intravenous contrast mediums or other injections, and vasovagal episodes (fainting). The risk of a trivial injury was 7 per thousand, and of a temporary disabling injury 400 per million. Temporary disabling injuries included 'reactions to adrenergic drugs', corneal abrasions, 'local injuries from needle insertion', fevers, nausea, assault by another participant, seizure after drug withdrawal, and an electrical burn under a pressure cuff. The one permanently disabling injury was a stroke 'that occurred three days after the subject participated in research on diabetes and hyperlipaemia, but the physician was not at all certain that the stroke was related to the research.'

6. Emotional

It is perhaps unremarkable that, when so little information has been recorded about the physical risks of research procedures, even less has been written about the emotional risks to children. Two studies suggest that these risks may often be underestimated. The first study was undertaken at Yale University over ten years ago in the early days of treatment of children with short stature with human growth hormone.[52] Schwartz and his colleagues started to prepare children for admission to a research unit at least six months before such admission was due. Children were included in all discussions with their parents, and were able to visit the unit prior to admission. During the research admission at least two interviews were conducted by a child psychiatrist, who found that, regardless of the careful preparation, none of the 17 children under the age of 11 showed any awareness that his admission had anything to do with research. Six of the 19 children aged over 11 years (and up to 17½ years) showed awareness that their admission had to do with research, and of these six, five 'showed symptoms of overwhelming anxiety'; two left the research unit after a few days refusing to continue in the research programme. Thus, the preparative efforts designed to reduce the anxiety felt by the child subjects of research had failed to do so.

A recent British study reported unexpected social and emotional problems during a randomized within-patient comparison of the effects of diet on diabetic control in 11 children.[11] The children had been invited to join the trial on the basis of four criteria – age over 10 years, ability of the children with their parents to give informed consent, stable family, and positive attitude to diabetic care – in order to exclude families that might find difficulty in coping with the trial. Subsequently it emerged that four families should not have been selected: the parents of one child had been separated for years, one boy was extremely distressed by the venepunctures, as was also the oldest subject, a 17-year-old girl. A 13-year-old girl turned out to have been falsifying her urine tests for months before the trial, and it became apparent that her father had had strong reservations about her joining the trial. During the trial, seven of the children suffered unexpected problems. One child's diabetes went out of control and he had to withdraw from the trial. Three children reported new or unexpected problems at school such as ketoacidotic vomiting during examinations. One child developed severe epigastric pain and another had severe chest pain; in neither case was any physical cause discovered. The conclusions drawn were 'that despite careful selection, children and adolescents in clinical trials will have social and emotional problems and these will be mainly unpredictable. Therefore, children and their families who are engaged in research will require continuing emotional support, and provision for the necessary support should perhaps be built into the design of such trials.'

It is important to remember the possible emotional consequences to a child merely of being in hospital. Some dramatic short-term consequences were shown by the early films of James Robertson, but other workers have examined effects in the longer term. Douglas[53] showed that a single hospital stay of less than one week's duration for children under the age of five had no adverse effects in general on emotional development in later childhood. On the other hand, multiple brief hospital admissions, and admissions of greater than one week in the first five years of life, were associated with an increased incidence of emotional problems in later years. These results, however, concerned children who had been admitted to hospital in an era of paediatric practice that had barely been affected by the recommendations of the Platt Report.[54] A recent report from New Zealand[55] concluded that in an enlightened paediatric setting, in which there were no limitations on parental visiting and ample provision for parents to stay overnight, there was little evidence to suggest that admission to hospital had any effect on a child's subsequent behaviour. The National Association for the Welfare of Children in Hospital undertook a survey in 1982[56] of all acute wards in England that nursed children up to the age of 16 years. This survey showed that only 49 per cent of such wards allowed unrestricted access by parents; in one region the figure was as low as 21 per cent. So the enlightened paediatric setting that prevents behavioural sequelae to hospital admission is not available in half the wards to which children are admitted. It must therefore be remembered that in many centres research that causes more frequent or longer stays in hospital may contribute to later emotional or behavioural problems.

In discussing the risks of research in child psychiatry, Graham[57] makes the point that it is extremely difficult to predict in advance the emotional risks to an individual child. 'A psychiatric interview, for example, in an epidemiological survey in which a child is asked among other items about his concerns, anxieties and fantasies could be seen, and indeed has been seen, either as a non-intrusive benign procedure involving negligible risk (compared for example to the everyday experience of exposure to insensitive criticism from parents, teachers and peers), or as a potentially highly disturbing event leading to prolonged distress because previously suppressed material is now exposed with little or no attempt to make it meaningful for the child.'

The information available about the emotional consequences to children of being research subjects is therefore inadequate for any formal risk estimation. The two studies mentioned above,[11,52] both of which were long-term studies of a chronic illness, provided evidence of severe emotional stress in 11 out of 47 subjects. Such emotional stress may often be an exacerbation of pre-existing stress rather than stress that has arisen *de novo*. It would be reasonable to conclude that long-term studies in children with chronic illness are likely to provoke emotional stress in a significant proportion of subjects. Other studies may provoke emotional stress in a less predictable fashion.

The foregoing has illustrated the possibilities and the difficulties in only one of the two elements of risk estimation: the calculation of the probability of a harm occurring. As we have already seen there are very considerable problems in quantifying the disutility of a given harm. There remain two parts of the process of risk assessment in proposals for research on children that should be considered before looking at some examples of risk/benefit analysis in practice. These are risk identification and risk perception.

Risk identification again

The risks identified so far are the relatively obvious ones of physical and emotional harms. But there are other risks that should in certain circumstances be considered in the overall risk/benefit analysis. The first of these are the risks to which a child is already exposed before entry into a research project. The Black Report,[58] for instance, has drawn attention to the fact that children in social class IV or V are already exposed to between five and seven times the risk of accidental death of children in social class I. Similarly, children in lower social classes are exposed to a much higher risk of chronic respiratory disease than children in social class I. It is known also that maternal depression may have a considerable influence on children's lives: the children of depressed mothers are twice as likely as the average to have accidents at home.[59] Behavioural disturbances are also much more common. Moreover, maternal depression in a random sample of women living in central London was strongly positively related to social class. Only 5 per cent of middle class women with children under the age of 6 living at home were depressed, while 42 per cent of working-class women in similar circumstances were depressed.[60] As previously suggested, children with pre-existing chronic illnesses may already be under considerable emotional strain; one study showed the presence of adverse psychosocial factors in the family background of 39 per cent of a group of diabetic children.[61]

A study performed on malnourished Nigerian children illustrates the need to consider carefully whether it is ethical to impose even a very small additional risk on children who are already greatly at risk.[62] The levels of antibodies to both types of Herpesvirus hominis – type I causes lesions such as cold sores, while type II causes genital herpes – were estimated in children aged 1 to 4 years, 16 of whom had marasmus and 37 of whom had kwashiorkor, two extreme forms of malnutrition. Five millilitres of blood were taken from each child subject, but only 0.5 ml was needed from each of the 64 well-nourished children who acted as controls. The study was undertaken to confirm a fairly obvious epidemiological point: that children who came from the very poor socioeconomic conditions in which marasmus and kwashiorkor can develop are predisposed to herpes virus infections. Since it is well known that such children are predisposed to a variety of bacterial infections and to other viral infections – measles in particular – the results of the study, showing that antibodies to the herpes viruses were more common in malnourished children than in well-nourished children, were hardly unexpected. Since this study was not designed in any way to be of therapeutic benefit one may ask whether the investigators were justified in confirming a minor epidemiological point by using children with life-threatening illnesses. It would also be of interest to know why it was necessary to take ten times as much blood from the malnourished children as from the well-nourished controls.

These examples illustrate the strength of the point put to the working group that some children, particularly those in social classes IV and V, are already exposed to such a degree of risk that it would be unacceptable to increase that degree of risk by adding to it the physical and emotional risks of being a research subject. This point is particularly important when it is considered together with some evidence from the United States that suggests that re-search subjects of lower social class tend to be in research projects of greater risk than subjects from higher social classes. Barber[63] found, in his survey of the control of research in the United States, that research projects with the possibility of considerable thera-peutic benefit to the subjects were most likely to be carried out on private patients, while projects of little or no therapeutic benefit were most likely to be carried out on patients who were welfare recipients. He also found the converse to be true: that projects in which the risks were relatively high compared to the possible benefits were twice as likely to be carried out on welfare recipients, compared to private patients, as projects with a more favourable risk/benefit analysis.

Other risks that a research ethics committee may need to consi-der are risks related to the investigator. It has already been shown that some research procedures are of greater risk when carried out by an inexperienced investigator than by someone who has been doing them for years. Dollery[64] has listed some of the problems that need to be considered by an ethics committee, and for the re-solution of many of which local knowledge will be essential. His list includes:

(1) Unwise enthusiasts
(2) Poorly trained staff
(3) Inadequate facilities
(4) Inaccurate data
(5) Dishonest interpretation
(6) Accidents
(7) Negligence.

Obviously, items (4) and (5) may not increase the physical risk to a subject, but they would suggest that subjects had been involved in a project under false pretences, so that it would be unethical to expose them to any risk at all.

Another aspect of the risks associated with investigators was revealed by Barber's study.[63] He assessed the performance of investigators working with human subjects in terms of the number of scientific papers published in the previous five years, the number of citations in the Science Citation Index to all papers published by the investigator in his three most highly cited years of work, and whether the investigator had been promoted to a rank in his institution that was commensurate with his achievements. These investigators were then asked to act as if they were a research ethics committee composed of a single member and to assess a number of hypothetical research problems; they were also asked to assess the projects that they were themselves conducting in terms of risk and benefit. Barber found that if investigators had not done well either in their local institution's competition for rewards or in terms of their recognition in the Science Citation Index, they were more likely than others to be involved in studies with less favourable risk/benefit ratios for the subjects, and were more likely to be permissive – i.e. permitting high risks or low benefits – in their assessment of the hypothetical proposals. This suggests that research ethics committees may sometimes need to assess the research record of investigators when considering their research proposals.

Risk perception

The final part of risk assessment that should be considered is the way in which researchers and lay people perceive the risks of research on children. A survey of chairmen of paediatric departments and directors of paediatric clinical research centres in the United States was reported in 1981.[65] The respondents were asked to assess the risk of performing various research procedures on children of different ages, and to state into which category of risk, defined in the report *Research involving children*,[66] the various risks fell. *Research involving children* was prepared by the US National Commission for the Protection of Human Subjects of Biomedical and Behavioral Research, and defined minimal risk as 'the probability and magnitude of physical or psychological harm that is normally encountered in the daily lives, or in the routine medical or psychological examination, of healthy children'. The report then uses two further categories of risk: 'a minor increase over minimal risk' and 'a greater than minor increase over minimal risk'. It seems reasonable to suppose that these three categories are essentially similar to the BPA's three categories of 'negligible', 'minimal', and 'more than minimal'.[1] It is regrettable, however, that 'minimal' should be used in two different ways, and that the British definition should be further from standard English usage. The American usage will be followed in the conclusions of this report.

The results of the risk perception study showed, rather surprisingly, that some respondents were willing to regard all the following procedures as being of minimal risk (American definition) at any age from new-born to 18 years old:

Venepuncture at: antecubital fossa (elbow)
                 femoral vein (groin)
                 external jugular vein (neck)
                 internal jugular vein (neck)
Arterial puncture
Tympanocentesis (puncture of the eardrum)
Punch biopsy of skin
Bone scan
Intramuscular injection of placebo

Arterial puncture, for instance, was regarded as being of minimal risk to new-born infants by 8 per cent, and of minimal risk to 12- to 18-year-olds by no less than 24 per cent of the respondents. It seems impossible to correlate this response with the previous evidence of a 39 per cent risk of minor complications even in adults. Fifty-five per cent of respondents thought punch biopsy of the skin to be of minimal risk to new-born infants, yet Cardon[51] reported a study in which scars developed after 40 out of 75 such biopsies. It is assumed that the bone scan referred to is what in Britain might be called a skeletal survey: the dose of radiation absorbed from such a survey approaches 5 mSv, particularly if views of the spine are required, at which level the risks, given earlier, are certainly greater than those generally accepted for medical procedures. Yet 55 per cent or more of the respondents thought the procedure to be of minimal risk even for new-born infants.

It would appear that the chief conclusion to be drawn from this survey of the perceptions of paediatricians and paediatric researchers is that they are unrealistically optimistic about the risks of research. Such a conclusion was also suggested, although not specifically stated, by Barber's study.[63] It accords too with the results of some assessments of the seriousness of various illnesses. Wyler and his colleagues[67] received replies to a questionnaire from 117 physicians and 141 lay people; the questionnaire asked the respondents to rate a list of illnesses according to their relative seriousness. The rank order correlation coefficient was 0.947, indicating a very high degree of correlation between the medical and the lay lists. Yet the lists contained some extraordinary results, showing that both doctors' and patients' perceptions of seriousness have little relation to the actual risk of death. Thus, strokes and heart attacks – two of the most common causes of death – were perceived as less serious than meningitis, multiple sclerosis, or uraemia; frigidity was thought to be more serious than pneumonia or appendicitis; and a slipped disc was rated as more serious than starvation! It is understandable that lay assessment of the seriousness of an illness such as meningitis may be influenced emotively by popular images of its horror that probably derive from a pre-antibiotic era. If, however, doctors' perceptions about diseases for which accurate mortality statistics are available can be so bizarre, it is difficult to suggest that their perceptions of the risks of research procedures are likely to be any more accurate.

Examples of risk/benefit analysis

It will be observed that no mention has been made of attempts to quantify benefit in research on children. This is because research projects have such a large variety of purposes and possible outcomes that no useful categorization appears possible. Since, in calculating benefit, one is trying to assess the utility of new knowledge, it is inevitable that the operation will be less a calculation and more a guesstimate. It seems more useful to attempt a couple of risk/benefit analyses on projects reported in British journals, one of which was a non-therapeutic research project and the other of which was therapeutic. While the assessment of potential benefit cannot be made much more precise, a numerical method will be suggested that might give some indication of the magnitude of benefit that would be required to justify a given risk.

Example 1. Liver biopsy

Previous mention was made of several reports in which liver biopsies had been performed. One such report is that of Nayak *et al.*[4] who investigated the livers of 29 children aged 2 months to 6 years, with a mean age of 1.6 years, who were siblings of patients with Indian childhood cirrhosis of the liver (ICC). The aetiology of this disease is unknown, but it has been observed that more than one child in a family may be afflicted even though there is no clear pattern of inheritance. A previously asymptomatic sibling of a child with ICC may later develop ICC himself, and it has been suggested that an inherited susceptibility to the disease may allow the disease to develop under the influence of some unknown agent.

Nayak's report gives no information about liver function tests in the 29 children, who are, however, described as being asymptomatic, but it does report normal biochemical findings in 2 children who acted as controls. The 29 children each had a percutaneous liver biopsy performed, while the two controls had a wedge biopsy of the liver taken at laparotomy for an unrelated condition, congenital megacolon. None of the 31 liver biopsies showed any significant abnormalities: a few 'mild and non-specific alterations within the range of the so-called "normal"' were all that were found.

The risks of percutaneous liver biopsy have been previously outlined, and are between 160 and 200 per million for death, and between 4 and 5.4 per thousand for a major complication. There was therefore in the whole study, involving 29 children, approximately a 15 per cent risk that a child would suffer a major complication. Had sequential statistical analysis been applied to the findings, a significant result would have been found after the performance of 7 biopsies, and a highly significant result after 10 biopsies. Thus, at least 19 of the children were exposed to the risks of liver biopsy unnecessarily. The ages of the children were such that considerable restraint, or more probably sedation, would have been required: otherwise the risk, for instance, of producing a pneumothorax would have been much higher than the figure given above for major complications. No mention however is made of this in the report.

Assessment of the possible benefit is difficult, since Nayak and his colleagues nowhere give any indication of what they thought that they might discover. The children were healthy with, it is presumed, normal hepatic biochemistry: thus, the procedure was not performed with any therapeutic intention towards its subjects. Normal hepatic biochemistry would also make unlikely any major change in liver histology. The study was therefore designed to examine children who were functionally and biochemically normal, in the hope that some abnormality might turn up. If that abnormality had been found, it was then possible that it might have provided a clue to the unknown agent that may precipitate the disease in a susceptible child. It is a truism of all scientific research that if one does not know what one is looking for, one is most unlikely to find it.

The definition of benefit adopted at the beginning of this chapter was that of the Royal Society, which included the statement: 'Expected benefit incorporates an estimate of the probability of achieving the gain.' If one attempts a reasonably optimistic estimate of the probability of a beneficial result from Nayak's study, one might start with the likelihood of finding abnormal biopsies. In asymptomatic children, presumed to have normal hepatic biochemistry, there is most unlikely to be a greater than 20 per cent chance of finding a significant histological abnormality. If such an abnormality were found, the chance in turn of its leading to a specific noxious agent is unlikely to be greater than 10 per cent. The chance of any noxious agent that was found being the specific precipitating factor in ICC might be as high as 50 per cent. When these chances are multiplied together, an optimistic estimate would be that there was a 1 per cent chance of finding significant new information that might help other children.

The only reasonable verdict on this risk/benefit analysis is that the subject children were exposed – most of them unnecessarily even within the aims of the study – to a high level of risk with no possibility of benefit to themselves, and only a very small chance of any benefit to other children in the future. In fact, the balance is so weighted against the subject children as to make this study quite unethical, regardless of the 'permission' that was obtained (it is not stated from whom).

An alternative approach to risk/benefit analysis is suggested by Rosser's scale of valuations of states of illness[14] referred to earlier in this chapter. She developed a scale giving a numerical value of states of illness each made up of one of eight degrees of disability and one of four degrees of distress. Her scale is one of several indicators of health status that have been developed in recent years and which were reviewed at a series of Social Science Research Council workshops;[68] unlike some indicators, it is potentially fairly straightforward to use in practice, as was shown by a DHSS economic adviser[69] in the field of resource allocation. Table 5.5 shows the values that she obtained from her 70 adult respondents and the definitions of distress and disability that she used: it is evident that the scale may not be entirely appropriate for use with children, but it will serve to illustrate a possible method of calculation.

The purpose of the calculation is to determine a total disutility, or utility, score for a particular project. The length of time for which each harm potentially caused by the research would last is multiplied by its valuation on the Rosser scale; the product is then

Table 5.5   Scale of valuations of states of illness

		Distress state			
		1	2	3	4
Disability					
state	1		1.00	2.00	6.67
	2	2.00	2.70	5.45	13.50
	3	4.00	5.53	8.75	17.50
	4	7.25	8.70	11.67	26.00
	5	10.85	13.03	20.00	60.00
	6	25.00	31.00	64.00	200.00
	7	64.50	87.20	200.00	497.14
	8	405.71			
	Death	200.00			

Distress states:	1	No Distress
	2	Mild distress
	3	Moderate distress
	4	Severe distress
Disability states:	1	No disability
	2	Slight social disability
	3	Severe social disability and/or slight impairment of performance at work
	4	Choice of work or performance at work very severely limited
	5	Unable to work or to continue education. Housewives only able to perform a few simple tasks.
	6	Confined to chair or wheelchair.
	7	Confined to bed.
	8	Unconscious.

multiplied by the probability that that harm would occur, so as to derive a disutility score for an individual subject for a particular harm. The disutility scores for each harm to which an individual might be exposed are then multiplied by the total number of subjects and added together to give a disutility score for the whole project.

In Nayak's study, for instance, each individual child was exposed to a risk of death or of severe complications for which the probabilities are known. If death had occurred then the length of time for which that harm lasted would be the loss of life expectancy of that child. Life expectancy at birth in India is 49 years,[70] but infant mortality is so high that the life expectancy of survivors of infancy aged 1 year is approximately 55 years. The average age of the children in Nayak's study was 1.6 years, so death would have caused a loss of life expectancy of 54.4 years. Death on the Rosser scale is given a score of 200. Therefore, the disutility score for an individual child, using days rather than years for the time-scale, would be

$$54.4 \times 365 \times 200 \times \frac{200}{1\,000\,000} \; ; \text{i.e. } 794.$$

Thus, the total disutility score for all subjects for the risk of death would be 23 026. A standard British textbook[70] recommends that, in toddlers, the procedure be carried out under general anaesthetic. The risk of death from a general anaesthetic was given earlier as 20 per million; if the liver biopsies in Nayak's study were performed under general anaesthetic, one should add 2303 to the total disutility score.

It is customary to keep children confined to bed for 24 hours after a liver biopsy; since it is likely that they would be in some distress, it is suggested that all the subjects would be in the Rosser scale's state 7,2 for one day. This would give a disutility score of 29×87.20, i.e. 2529.

The serious complications that might arise from a liver biopsy are intraperitoneal bleeding or infection, pneumothorax or biliary peritonitis. It is suggested that, were one of these complications to arise, the child would be in the Rosser scale's state 7,4 for perhaps 4 days, and in state 6,3 for about ten days. Serious complications would, therefore, give a disutility score of

$$29 \times \tfrac{5.4}{1000} \times (497 \times 4 + 64 \times 10) = 412.$$

Thus, for those risks whose probabilities are known approximately, one could predict that Nayak's study would produce a total disutility score of 23 026+2303+2529+412 =28 270. If one's purpose in risk/benefit analysis were merely to ensure that risks and benefits were evenly balanced, then one would wish to see benefits arise from a research project to the same numerical value as the risks. In this example one would, for instance, wish the project to return to normality children who would otherwise have been in Rosser's state 1,2, scoring 1.00, for a total of 28 270 days. Alternatively one would wish to see an increase in life expectancy of $\tfrac{28\ 270}{200}$ days.

However, it is widely accepted that such an equal balance in non-therapeutic research would impose far too great a burden on the research subjects. For the sake of argument, it is suggested that in such a non-therapeutic research project, one should be able to predict benefits to at least ten times the value of the risks. In the case of Nayak's study, therefore, one would wish to be able to predict a utility score of 282 700. Since the probability of any benefit has already been calculated as being only 1 per cent, it is suggested that one needs to be able to demonstrate that the benefits, that would arise from the study if a predisposing factor to ICC were found, should be assessed at a utility score of 28 270 000. If the study benefits were truly life-saving, then such a score would in fact be easy to achieve, since the saving of a toddler's life, according to this scale, produces a utility score of 54.4×365×200, i.e. approximately 4 000 000. Thus, one would only need to restore 8 toddlers who would otherwise have died to perfect health to satisfy the requirement. Since ICC is a disease which normally follows an inexorable course to death, it is more likely that the benefits might just have been a temporary improvement in the condition of children with the disease. If, for instance, a child who would normally have been in Rosser's state 5,3 were returned for one year to state 3,1, i.e. from severe disability with moderate distress to moderate disability with no distress, then that benefit would represent a utility score of 365×(20.0−4.00) = 5840. In that case, one would need to be able to give that benefit to almost 5000 children with the illness in order to satisfy the risk/benefit requirements.

Such mathematical risk/benefit analysis is obviously still at a crude stage of development. With the ever-increasing sophistication of health indicators it is suggested, however, that such analysis may offer research ethics committees and others the possibility of more appropriate ethical assessment of projects – particularly those which are non-therapeutic or appear to carry a high level of risk. If such a scoring system proves in practice to be of value, then members of research ethics committees such as statisticians and those involved in research will have to be prepared to help lay members of the committees in its use.

Example 2. Penicillin allergy

An investigation by Chandra *et al.*[71] of 300 children considered to have had adverse reactions to penicillin provides an example of the possibilities of risk/benefit analysis in therapeutic research projects. The incidence of hypersensitivity reactions to penicillin ranges from 0.7 to 10 per cent in different reports. Such reactions range from mild skin rashes to serum sickness, anaphylaxis, and death. The risk of anaphylaxis following administration of penicillin is between 150 and 400 per million. The risk of death from anaphylaxis due to penicillin is 20 per million, and, worldwide, there are at least 300 deaths per annum.[72] Anaphylaxis is a sudden loss of blood pressure with bronchospasm as in severe asthma, and loss of fluid from the circulating blood volume. Normally, any reaction to penicillin is taken as a contraindication to its further use in the patient. Nevertheless, it is an extremely useful antibiotic, and so Chandra and his co-workers studied whether all the children in a group said to have had reactions to penicillin were in fact hypersensitive to it.

Penicillin forms various breakdown products when given to humans, one of which (penicilloyl polylysine) is called the 'major determinant' of penicillin since so many hypersensitivity reactions appear to be caused by it. Other breakdown products, and sodium benzylpenicillin G itself, are called the 'minor determinants' since they cause reactions less frequently. The severity of a reaction to penicillin or its major or minor determinants is not dose-related, and can be as severe for the minor as for the major determinants. The test procedure used by Chandra was to perform first a scratch or prick test either with the major or the minor determinants of penicillin. If after 10 minutes there was no reaction, he went on to give an intradermal injection of 0.03 ml of each test substance; the test was read as positive if there was a weal at least 3 mm larger than that of a saline control injection after at least 20 minutes. A

0.1 mg dose of sodium benzylpenicillin was injected as part of the minor determinant mixture, compared with an average daily dose for a 7-year-old child of 600 mg. Blood was also obtained from each child to measure the amount of a specific antibody, penicilloyl-specific IgE, by the radioallergosorbent test, or RAST. Both the skin test and the blood test are well-recognized as being suitable for diagnosing penicillin hypersensitivity, although neither test is totally reliable.

The frequency of positive tests – by skin reaction or the presence of antibody determined by RAST, or both – was 19 per cent. The validity of the tests was confirmed in two ways. Of 56 children with negative tests only 2 produced a mild skin rash on 'subsequent drug challenge'; it is not recorded whether this drug challenge arose because an infection was treated with penicillin in each of the 56 children, or whether they were given a test dose of the drug. The other validation of the tests arose because the 'inadvertent administration of penicillin in 5 patients with positive tests resulted in rapid generalized urticaria in each'.[71]

There appear to be two principal sources of risk in this study: the first, venepuncture, has a risk of fatality of less than one per million. No indication is given of the ages of the children, so no comment can be made about the risks of non-fatal physical injury or emotional distress. The second hazard is the performance of skin tests. All the children had already had a reaction to penicillin, and were therefore in the group – 0.7 to 10 per cent of all children – that includes children who develop anaphylaxis. Thus, while the risk of anaphylaxis to all children is 150 to 400 per million, the risk to these children of anaphylaxis following a further dose of penicillin must lie between 1.5 per thousand at the lowest, and 57 per thousand at the highest estimate. Similarly, the risk of death for the child subjects of this study is increased and lies in the range 0.2 to 2.8 per thousand. What is not certain is whether the risk of a severe reaction is as great for the small amounts of major and minor determinants used as for a normal dose. Goodman and Gilman[72] comment: 'It must be stressed that fatal episodes of anaphylaxis have followed the ingestion of very small doses of this antibiotic or skin testing with minute quantities of the drug.' For present purposes, it will be suggested that the risks are at the lower ends of the two ranges: i.e. in this study the risk of anaphylaxis was 1.5 per thousand, and the risk of death was 0.2 per thousand.

In assessing the potential benefits of this study, as they might have been specified before it started, one may distinguish between benefits to the subjects and benefits to children in general. The principal potential benefit to each child subject would be to know for certain whether or not he was allergic to penicillin. Benefits to other children would only accrue if the results of the study were so striking that they led to a change in the pattern of prescribing of penicillin to children, a pattern which had developed over a period of thirty years prior to this study.

The most important benefit to an individual child would be to know that he has a penicillin allergy since he and his family could then avoid the potentially fatal administration of penicillin in the future. In this study, 57 children had positive tests, although only 33 had both a positive skin test and a positive blood test. Five of these children were subsequently given penicillin and all developed accelerated urticaria. To paraphrase Oscar Wilde, to give one allergic child penicillin may be regarded as a misfortune; to do it twice looks like carelessness. It is suggested that to do it five times indicates that this study included no mechanism for warning parents and their children about positive allergy results; certainly there is no mention of, for instance, the issuing of warning cards, or of any other system for avoiding penicillin in the allergic children, in the published report. In considering the potential benefits of this study, therefore, one must exclude any benefit to individual children of being found to be allergic to penicillin since this information was neither communicated to the subjects nor acted upon.

The other possible benefit to an individual child would be to know that he was no longer allergic to penicillin, or else never had been, and that it would be safe in future for him to have penicillin. Although penicillin remains the drug of choice in some streptococcal infections, there are many alternative antibiotics available: occasions on which penicillin would be the only effective antibiotic are extremely uncommon. There would certainly be occasions when it might be cheaper and simpler to give a child penicillin and there are conditions in which long-term treatment with penicillin is needed. In the latter case, however, it would be possible to do the tests for allergy at the time that long-term treatment became necessary. The probability of this potential benefit actually becoming useful therefore seems likely to be rather low.

Benefits to children other than the subjects might arise if the study produced generalizable information that altered the prescribing policy summed up by Laurence: 'when there is even a suspicion of penicillin allergy the drug is best totally avoided *and the patient warned*' (his emphasis).[73] Such a change in policy might result, if all the children were shown to have a penicillin allergy, in which case warnings about the avoidance of penicillin after any sort of reaction to it could be redoubled, or the study might show that none of the children had evidence of an allergy to penicillin, so that the precautions might be relaxed slightly. Neither such result would have been at all likely, however, since they do not accord with the very substantial body of knowledge available before the study started. It would probably be wildly over-generous to suggest that there would be even one chance in a million of such a result. A third possible benefit to other children would arise if there were shown to be a definite point, a certain number of years after the most recent adverse reaction to penicillin, after which all traces of penicillin allergy had disappeared. Such a result is slightly more likely than the other two, since it is known that evidence of allergy declines the longer the time since the last dose of penicillin. But there have also been cases of adverse reactions to penicillin occurring many years after previous such reactions.

There is such a wealth of experience in the use of penicillin that the chances of this study having found any information of benefit to children other than the subjects seem extremely small. There were two possible benefits to the subjects: one benefit did not happen because of failures in communication, and the other benefit was really quite small. On the other hand, the risks of death or anaphylaxis were substantial since the study population (300) was quite large. Thus, although at first sight the study appears to be quite straightforward and to offer some chance of benefit to the subjects, closer examination suggests that the risks outweigh the benefits by a substantial margin.

As in the previous example, of liver biopsy, it is possible to try to quantify this risk/benefit analysis by calculating disutility and utility scores using Rosser's scale of valuations of states of illness. The Canadian children in this study might be expected to have, on average, a life expectancy of 73 years; their ages are not given, so an arbitrary average age of 10 years will be assumed. Thus, were a child to die, the loss of life expectancy would be $(73-10) \times 365$ days; the lower end of the range calculated for the risk of death was 0.2 per thousand, and the Rosser scale gives a value of 200 for death. So the disutility score for the risk of death would be

$$(73-10) \times 365 \times 200 \times 300 \times \frac{0.2}{1000}, \text{ i.e. } 275\ 940.$$

The disutility of anaphylaxis has both acute and chronic elements. Initially it is an extremely serious illness causing great distress; if not treated immediately it can lead to death, or can cause brain damage as a result of a drastic drop in the supply of oxygen to the brain. If treated successfully it often progresses to another form of allergic disease, serum sickness, which may take a week or more to clear up, with substantial disability from skin rashes and joint pain before it does so. It is suggested that a child suffering anaphylaxis would be in Rosser's state of illness 7,4 for one day, followed by state 7,3 for one day, then state 6,3 for three days and would finally be in state 6,2 for a further three days. Using the valuations for these states and the risk of anaphylaxis of 1.5 per thousand, the estimated disutility score for acute anaphylaxis would be

$$(497.14+200.00+3\times64.00+3\times31.00)\times300\times\tfrac{1.5}{1000}, \text{ i.e. } 442.$$

The figures previously used suggest that when anaphylaxis occurs, between one patient in seven and one in twenty dies; for the sake of argument, it will be suggested that one patient in twenty is left with residual brain damage that leaves the patient in Rosser's state 4,2. The disutility score for the long-term effects of anaphylaxis would then be

$$63\times365\times8.70\times300\times\tfrac{1.5}{1000}\times\tfrac{1}{20}, \text{ i.e. } 4501.$$

The total disutility score for this study would therefore be 280 883.

The earlier discussion of benefit showed that the only likely benefits were those which accrued to the 243 subjects found not to be allergic to penicillin. The most likely reason for needing to use long-term penicillin treatment would be in the prophylaxis of rheumatic carditis. The upper end of the range of figures for its incidence in a population such as that of the penicillin allergy study is 150 per 100 000. Prophylaxis is usually continued for about 25 years. If during that period, a child who might otherwise have been in the Rosser state 4,3 were kept normal by the prophylaxis, then the utility score for one child would be $25\times365\times11.67$. For this study, then, the utility score would be

$$\tfrac{243\times150}{100\ 000}\times25\times365\times11.67, \text{ i.e. } 38\ 815$$

Apart from streptococcal infections, penicillin remains the antibiotic of choice mostly for infections that are quite rare in Canada, such as anthrax, tetanus, and gas gangrene. The utility of penicillin to the 243 non-allergic children will therefore be estimated for the treatment of acute infections by reference to streptococcal infections, which most commonly will be upper respiratory infections. It is suggested that, in such an infection, a person treated with penicillin would be in Rosser's state 4,4 for one day only and would then revert to state 2,2 for three days before returning to normality; the total score for four days would then be 26.00+3×2.70, i.e. 39.10. Had it not been known that the patient was not allergic to penicillin, an alternative, perhaps less effective, antibiotic would have been used, leading to two days each in states 4,4, 3,3, and 2,2 before a return to normality. The total score for the six days would be 2×(26.00+8.75+2.70), i.e. 74.90. So the use of penicillin in an acute upper respiratory illness might reduce the total illness score by 74.9−34.1, i.e. 40.8. If one assumed that on average each of the 243 children would avail themselves of this advantage ten times during the rest of their lives – probably a considerable overestimate – the total utility of this benefit would be

243×10×40.8, i.e. 99 144.

By using slightly optimistic calculations one may therefore arrive at a possible utility score for this study of 38 815+99 144, a total of 137 959. This is, however, just under half the disutility score calculated on the basis of the risks of death and anaphylaxis. The intuitive assessment that the risks of the study appeared to outweigh the benefits is therefore confirmed by estimation of the disutility and utility scores. It should be noted that the study report states: 'Informed consent was obtained from the parents. The study protocol had been approved by the Human Experimentation Committees of the hospital and the university.'[71]

Conclusions

These two examples, both of an intuitive and of an arithmetical approach to risk/benefit analysis, have been given in order to illustrate the difficulties facing any research ethics committee or investigator who tries to make an honest appraisal of the risks and benefits of proposed research projects. It is hoped that they may be seen as representative of the not infrequent research projects on children that do not have an obvious or substantial therapeutic intention to the subjects of the research and therefore require careful review by research ethics committees. Some projects will hold out the prospect of considerably greater benefit to other children than the two examples given. What these examples tend to suggest is that clinical research on children is still carried out in which the researchers have not adequately considered questions that must be answered before undertaking research:

(i)　Is the right question being asked?
(ii)　Is this study the right way to answer it?
(iii)　If the study does provide an answer, will it be worth knowing?

It is vital that the answer to all these questions be in the affirmative, because it is not ethical to carry out research that is not scientifically valid.

There is a more general problem about the assessment of risk and benefit that depends on the limitations in our means of measuring them. This has best been expressed by Dollery: 'We also know, from such studies as have been done, that the benefits that are achieved in the ordinary practice of medicine from the use of therapeutic procedures are usually less than are achieved from using the same procedures in randomized controlled trials, because they are applied with less skill to less appropriately chosen patients, and often with less persistence. Thus, one can say that the benefits are less than we believe. On the other hand, it is clear that there are still undocumented risks of treatment, whether by drugs, surgery or investigative procedures, so that the risks are greater than we know. I believe one of the problems that we suffer is that we have over claimed the benefits of treatment in the past.'[74]

The examples of risk/benefit analysis given indicate that, with care and persistence, it may become possible to undertake quite a full analysis of many projects, although it will be difficult to exclude value judgements entirely. The evidence presented of the inaccuracies in investigators' perceptions of risk suggests that it is important to work towards an arithmetical categorization of risk and away from such categories as negligible, minimal, minor increase over minimal, and so forth, which are impossible to define and rely heavily on perceptions of risk, particularly those of the professionals involved. For the present, however, it is necessary to use such categories and to try to relate them to known risks.

Table 5.6 Risk equivalents

British definition[1]	Negligible	Minimal	More than minimal.
American definition[66]	Minimal	Minor increase over minimal	Greater than minor increase over minimal.
Risk of death	less than 1 per million	1 to 100 per million	Greater than 100 per million.
Risk of major complication	less than 10 per million	10 to 1000 per million	Greater than 1000 per million.
Risk of minor complication	less than 1 per thousand	1 to 100 per thousand	Greater than 100 per thousand.

One attempt to find equivalence between different scales of risk and the statistical probabilities of certain adverse events is shown in Table 5.6. Obviously, such a table does not answer all the problems of risk assessment. A precise distinction between the degrees of harm that constitute minor and major complications will always be difficult to achieve. Nevertheless, many harms will be easy to classify: major haemorrhage, biliary peritonitis, a convulsion after drug withdrawal, or septicaemia would all be major complications, while short-lived pain or tenderness, small bruises or scars, and fainting would, of themselves, be minor complications (fainting might, however, lead to a major complication: head injury). The decision as to where the dividing line between two categories of probability should lie will also be open to argument. The suggestion, for instance, that a risk of a major complication of up to 10 per million should be minimal (American definition) is a compromise: doctors may ignore yet larger risks, while lay people probably do not ignore a risk of that magnitude. These problems illustrate also the difficulties inherent in the attempt to include both the probability and magnitude of a harm in a three point scale of risk, as used in both the American and British guidelines.

It is worth briefly relating the figures used in Table 5.6 to the risks of particular procedures collated earlier in this chapter. The risk figures for major complications or death for most of the practical procedures lie in the category 'greater than minor increase over minimal'. So procedures such as lung biopsy, liver biopsy, arterial puncture, and cardiac catheterization are all classified as being of greater than a minor increase over minimal risk. While such a conclusion might offend the perceptions of a few doctors, it seems likely to be in accord with most lay perceptions. By this classification, also, the overall risks of non-therapeutic research as shown by Cardon's survey[51] would lie in the category 'minor increase over minimal' for both major and minor complications. It seems perfectly acceptable to subject adults, who have given informed consent, to such a level of risk. After a long debate, the working group agreed unanimously, however, that it was not acceptable to subject children, for whom only a proxy consent was available, to even a minor increase over minimal risk in non-therapeutic research. In other words, non-therapeutic research on children, regardless of possible benefits, can only be undertaken ethically if the risks of the procedures involved are in the 'minimal' category. It should be noted that although there are no precise risk figures available for collecting a sample of venous blood, the scarcity of anecdotes of harm arising from this procedure compared to the frequency with which such blood samples are collected suggests that it lies in the 'minimal' risk category.

Finally, it is important to remember that it is the perception of a risk formed by the patient, or the patient's proxy, that is of overriding importance compared with the investigator's perception of the risk. Nevertheless, the patient's, or his proxy's, perceptions will in practice depend on the information given to him by the investigator. There is therefore a considerable onus on the investigator to be able to distinguish what is known objectively about a risk from his own perception of it.

References

1. British Paediatric Association. Guidelines to aid ethical committees considering research involving children. *Archs Dis. Childh.* **55,** 75–7 (1980).
2. Royal Society Study Group. *Risk assessment.* Royal Society, London (1983).
3. Rowe, W. D. *An anatomy of risk.* John Wiley, New York (1977).
4. Nayak, N. C., Marwaha, N., Kalra, V., Roy, S., and Ghai, O. P. The liver in siblings of patients with Indian childhood cirrhosis: a light and electron microscopic study. *Gut* **22,** 295–300 (1981).
5. Lichtenstein, P. K., Heubi, J. E., Daugherty, C. C., Farrell, M. K., Sokol, R. J., Rothbaum, R. J., Suchy, F. J., and Balistreri, W. F. Grade I Reye's syndrome. *New Engl. J. Med.* **309,** 133–9 (1983).
6. Scotto, J., Hadchouel, M., Hery, C., Alvarez, F., Yvart, J., Tiollais, P., Bernard, O., and Brechot, C. Hepatitis B virus DNA in children's liver diseases: detection by blot hybridisation in liver and serum. *Gut* **24,** 618–24 (1983).
7. Work Group XII of the National Institute of Arthritis, Metabolism and Digestive Diseases Evaluation Effort on the Future of Digestive Disease Research. Human experimentation in digestive disease research. *Gastroenterology* **69,** 1165–82 (1975).
8. McKay, R. J. Diagnosis and treatment: risks of obtaining samples of venous blood in infants. *Pediatrics* **38,** 906–8 (1966).
9. Raghuprasad, P. K. Venipuncture and cardiac arrest (letter). *J. Am. Med. Assoc.* **241,** 134–5 (1979).
10. Karp, G., Robert, N., and Papish, S. Infection from finger sticks in leukopenic patients (letter). *Ann. internal Med.* **95,** 392–3 (1981).
11. Kinmonth, A. L., Lindsay, M. K. M., and Baum, J. D. Social and emotional complications in a clinical trial among adolescents with diabetes mellitus. *Br. med. J.* **286,** 952–4 (1983).
12. Schimmel, E. M. The hazards of hospitalization. *Ann. internal Med.* **60,** 100–10 (1964).
13. Department of Transport. *Highways economics Note No. 1: Road accident costs 1981.* Department of Transport, London (1982).
14. Rosser, R., and Kind, P. A scale of valuations of states of illness: is there a social consensus? *Int. J. Epidemiol.* **7,** 347–58 (1978).
15. Council for Science and Society. *The acceptability of risks.* Barry Rose, London (1977).
16. Ashby, E. *Reconciling man with the environment,* pp.69–70. Oxford University Press, London (1978).
17. Card, W. I., and Mooney, G. H. What is the monetary value of a human life? *Br. med. J.* **2,** 1627–9 (1977).
18. Kletz, T. A. What risks should we run? *New Scient.* **74,** 320–2 (1977).
19. Pochin, E. E. Risk and medical ethics. *J. med. Ethics* **8,** 180–4 (1982).
20. ——. Occupational and other fatality risks. *Community Hlth* **6,** 2–13 (1974).
21. Nicholson, R. H. Can deafness be prevented in full-bore shooters? *Natn Rifle Assoc. J.* **LXII**(1), 20–2 and **LXII**(2), 29 (1983).

22. Central Statistical Office. *Social trends 15*. HMSO, London (1985).
23. Knox, E. G. Negligible risks to health. *Community Hlth* **6**, 244–51 (1975).
24. Chief Medical Officer of the DHSS. *On the state of the public health, 1971*. HMSO, London (1972).
25. Pochin, E. E. Quantification of risk in medical procedures. *Proc. R. Soc.* **A 376**, 87–101 (1981).
26. Department of Health and Social Security. *Whooping cough: Reports from the Committee on Safety of Medicines and the Joint Committee on Vaccination and Immunisation*. HMSO, London (1981).
27. Silverstein, A. M. *Pure politics and impure science*. Johns Hopkins University Press, Baltimore (1981).
28. Young, M. E. J. *Radiological physics* (3rd edn). H. K. Lewis, London (1983).
29. Stewart, A. The carcinogenic effects of low level radiation. A re-appraisal of epidemiologist's methods and observations. *Health Phys.* **24**, 223–240 (1973).
30. Girdwood, R. H. Death after taking medicaments. *Br. med. J.* **1**, 501–4 (1974).
31. Department of Health, Education and Welfare. *Report of the Secretary's Commission on Medical Malpractice* No. 0S-73-89. DHEW, Washington DC (1973).
32. Rodin, J. *Will this hurt? Preparing children for hospital and medical procedures*. Royal College of Nursing, London (1983).
33. Smith, M. Taking blood from children causes no more than minimal harm. *J. med. Ethics* **11**, 127–31 (1985).
34. Mortensen, J. D. Clinical sequelae from arterial needle puncture, cannulation, and incision. *Circulation* **XXXV**, 1118–23 (1967).
35. Gillies, I. D. S., Morgan, M., Sykes, M. K., Brown, A. E., and Jones, N. O. The nature and incidence of complications of peripheral arterial puncture. *Anaesthesia* **34**, 506–9 (1979).
36. Rudolph, A. M. Complications occurring in infants and children. *Circulation*, Suppl. III to vols XXXVII and XXXVIII, 59–66 (1968).
37. Varghese, P. J., Celermajer, J., Izukawa, T., Haller, J. A., and Rowe, R. D. Cardiac catheterization in the newborn: experience with 100 cases. *Pediatrics* **44**, 24–9 (1969).
38. Miller, G. A. H. Congenital heart disease in the first week of life. *Br. Heart J.* **36**, 1160–6 (1974).
39. Allison, D. J. and Hemingway, A. P. Percutaneous needle biopsy of the lung. *Br. med. J.* **282**, 875–8 (1981).
40. Pearce, J. M. S. Hazards of lumbar puncture. *Br. med. J.* **285**, 1521–2 (1982).
41. Fischer, G. W., Brenz, R. W., Alden, E. R., and Beckwith, J. B. Lumbar punctures and meningitis. *Am. J. Dis. Childh.* **129**, 590–2 (1975).
42. Teele, D. W., Dashefsky, B., Rakusan, T., and Klein, J. O. Meningitis after lumbar puncture in children with bacteremia. *New Engl. J. Med.* **305**, 1079–81 (1981).
43. Petersdorf, R. G., Swarner, D. R., and Garcia, M. Studies on the

pathogenesis of meningitis. II. Development of meningitis during pneumococcal bacteremia. *J. clin. Invest.* **41**, 320–7 (1962).
44. Schreiner, R. L. and Kleiman, M. B. Incidence and effect of traumatic lumbar puncture in the neonate. *Devl Med. & Child Neurol.* **21**, 483–7 (1979).
45. Zamchek, N. and Klausenstock, O. Liver Biopsy – II. The risk of needle biopsy. *New Engl. J. Med.* **249**, 1062–9 (1953).
46. Westaby, D., MacDougall, B. R. D., and Williams, R. Liver biopsy as a day-case procedure: selection and complications in 200 consecutive patients. *Br. med. J.* **281**, 1331–2 (1980).
47. —— and Williams, R. Liver biopsy as a day-case procedure (letter). *Br. med. J.* **282**, 478 (1981).
48. Knauer, C. M. Percutaneous biopsy of the liver as a procedure for outpatients. *Gastroenterology* **74**, 101–2 (1978).
49. Cooksley, W. G. E., Anaphylaxis to bromosulfophthalein. *Med. J. Aust.* **2**, 257–8 (1971).
50. Zarafonetis, C. J. D., Riley, P. A., Willis, P. W., Power, L. H., Werbelow, J., Farhat, L., Beckwith, W., and Marks, B. H. Clinically significant adverse effects in a Phase I testing program. *Clin. Pharmacol. & Ther.* **24**, 127–32 (1978).
51. Cardon, P. V., Dommel, F. W., Trumble, R. R. Injuries to research subjects. A survey of investigators. *New Engl. J. Med.* **295**, 650–4 (1976).
52. Schwartz, A. H. Children's concepts of research hospitalization. *New Engl. J. Med.* **287**, 589–92 (1972).
53. Douglas, J. W. B. Early hospital admissions and later disturbances of behaviour and learning. *Devl Med. & Child Neurol.* **17**, 456–80 (1975).
54. Ministry of Health. Central Health Services Council. *The welfare of children in hospital.* HMSO, London (1959).
55. Shannon, F. T., Fergusson, D. M., and Dimond, M. E. Early hospital admissions and subsequent behaviour problems in 6 year olds. *Archs Dis. Childh.* **59**, 815–19 (1984).
56. Thornes, R. Parental access and family facilities in children's wards in England. *Br. med. J.* **287**, 190–2 (1983).
57. Graham, P. J. Ethics and child psychiatry. In *Psychiatric ethics* (eds S. Bloch and P. Chodoff) pp.235–54. Oxford University Press, Oxford (1981).
58. Working Group on Inequalities in Health (Chairman: Sir D. Black). Report: *Inequalities in health.* DHSS, London (1980).
59. Brown, G. W. and Harris, T. *Social origins of depression.* Tavistock, London (1978).
60. ——, Ni Bhrolchain, M., and Harris, T. Social class and psychiatric disturbance among women in an urban population. *Sociology* **9**, 225–54 (1975).
61. Gath, A., Smith, M. A., and Baum, J. D. Emotional, behavioural, and educational disorders in diabetic children. *Archs Dis. Childh.* **55**, 371–5 (1980).
62. Johnson, A. O. K., Salimonn, L. S., and Osunkoya, B. O.

Antibodies to *Herpes virus hominis* types 1 and 2 in malnourished Nigerian children. *Archs Dis. Childh.* **56**, 45–8 (1981).
63. Barber, B., Lally, J. J., Makarushka, J. L., and Sullivan, D. *Research on human subjects: problems of social control in medical experimentation*, pp.53–7. Transaction Books, New Brunswick, NJ (1979).
64. Dollery, C. T. Clinical pharmacology. In *Ethical committees for clinical research: Report of a symposium*, p.127. Medico-Pharmaceutical Forum, London (1982).
65. Janofsky, J. and Starfield, B. Assessment of risk in research on children. *J. Pediat.* **98**, 842–6 (1981).
66. National Commission for the Protection of Human Subjects of Biomedical and Behavioral Research. *Research involving children;* Report and recommendations: 77-0004. DHEW, Washington DC (1977).
67. Wyler, A. R., Masuda, M., and Holmes, T. H. Seriousness of Illness Rating Scale. *J. Psychosom. Res.* **11**, 363–74 (1968).
68. Culyer, A. J. (ed.). *Health indicators.* Martin Robertson, Oxford (1983).
69. Teeling Smith, G. (ed.). *Measuring the social benefits of medicine.* Office of Health Economics, London (1983).
70. Forfar, J. O. and Arneil, G. C. (ed.) *Textbook of paediatrics* (3rd edn), p.1953. Churchill Livingstone, Edinburgh (1984).
71. Chandra, R. K., Joglekar, S. A., and Tomas, E. Penicillin allergy: anti-penicillin IgE antibodies and immediate hypersensitivity skin reactions employing major and minor determinants of penicillin. *Archs Dis. Childh.* **55**, 857–60 (1980).
72. Goodman Gilman, A., Goodman, L. S., Rall, T. W., and Murad, F. *The pharmacological basis of therapeutics* (7th edn), pp.1134–6. Macmillan, New York (1985).
73. Laurence, D. R. *Clinical pharmacology* (4th edn), p.7.36. Churchill Livingstone, Edinburgh (1973).
74. Dollery, C. T. Summary and conclusions. In *Risk-benefit analysis in drug research: proceedings of an international symposium* (ed. J. F. Cavalla), pp.186–7. MTP Press, Lancaster (1981).

6

Children and the law

In addition to any ethical guidelines, there are also legal provisions which circumscribe the conduct of research on children. The State is concerned to protect the interests of children in most circumstances. This concern is the greater when another intends to invade the physical integrity of a child, or to expose the child to the risk of harm. Indeed, the interests of children in such circumstances are taken so seriously that it is thought proper to use the law as the appropriate means of protecting them. By having recourse to law, the State is indicating that it is not content to leave provisions for the protection and welfare of the child to less formal social regulation, whether by agreement among the medical profession or among any other professional group or, *a fortiori*, by agreement between parents or between parents and doctors.

It cannot, therefore, sensibly be asserted that the law has no place in the subtle and complex relationship between doctor, parent, and child. The law is involved and will remain so. To argue otherwise is to suggest that Parliament ought to exempt one particular group, the medical profession, from the ordinary provisions of the law and thereby grant them immunity from any form of redress or sanction. That said, of course, it must be conceded that while it can be answered with certainty that the law is involved, it cannot be said with certainty what the law requires. There is an unfortunate lack of precision in the law. This means that doctors, parents, and children may not know whether a proposed course of action is lawful or not. It also means that legal advisers will tend to err on the side of caution and counsel against that which cannot, with a high degree of certainty, be said to be lawful. They will do this for the very good reason that thereby they avoid exposing clients to possible prosecution or civil claims for damages. But the danger is that such an approach may have a 'chilling effect' on research or innovation, some of which can only be done on children.

It must follow that while the doctor, the researcher, the parents, and others must accept the appropriateness of legal regulation, they are entitled to law which is not only sensitive to the various interests but is also relatively clear.

In the context of research on children, the lawyer is concerned principally with two questions: *who* can consent, and *to what* may that person consent? In the subsequent analysis, only the law of England and Wales will be considered.

Who may consent?

The law reinforces the commitment of medical ethics to respect for autonomy, by providing that a doctor may not ordinarily treat or touch a person without that person's consent. Failure to observe this basic legal principle will expose the doctor to a civil action for damages in the torts of battery or negligence and to a criminal prosecution for, at least, assault. Any consent is only real or valid if it is given voluntarily and free from pressure or duress, and after appropriate information about any risks, real or potential, of the procedure has been given. The amount of information which the doctor has to give to a person is, according to the most recent case law, particularly the case of *Chatterton* v. *Gerson,* (1981) QB 432, that which a reasonable member of the medical profession would give to a patient in the particular circumstances. It will be clear that such a standard tends to undermine the law's commitment to autonomy because it substitutes what doctors think ought to be told for what the person may wish to know. Some courts in other common law jurisdictions, such as Canada and New Zealand as well as in the United States, have rejected this approach. They have adopted the standard of what the reasonable patient would wish to know, which is a compromise between a standard determined by the medical profession and one which would require that the doctor respond to the particular and perhaps idiosyncratic or unusual needs of the patient. (See Robertson, 'Informed consent to medical treatment' (1981) 97 LQR 102.) It is possible that English law will move in this direction in due course, although there is no clear sign of that happening at present. (The House of Lords' decision in *Sidaway* v. *Governors of the Royal Bethlem Hospital and the Maudsley Hospital and others,* [1985] 1 All ER 643 may represent some movement, albeit not a great deal.) The importance of considering the information which the doctor is obliged in law to pass on, lies in the fact that it is important to determine first, whether the patient is being exposed to treatment only or to some form of clinical research; and, secondly, whether the person to be informed is the patient, or research subject, or is someone such as a parent consenting on his behalf. It seems certain (and there is Canadian legal authority to this effect: *Halushka* v. *University of Saskatchewan* (1965) 53 DLR (2nd)436) that the doctor is under an obligation to give more information to a patient who is undergoing research rather than treatment; and, it is submitted, it may be necessary to give even more information where the consent to be given is a proxy consent. This is because, as will be seen, someone purporting to give consent on another's behalf may be subject to greater limits as to what he can consent to than if he were to be consenting for himself. In this case it would follow that the doctor must give all that relevant information which would allow the person consenting properly to exercise his responsibilities.

The law's commitment to respect for a person's autonomy means that any consent (or refusal of consent) is legally valid, and therefore may be acted on, only if the person involved is capable of acting autonomously, or is, in legal language, competent. If the person purporting to give valid consent is not legally competent then, of course, the doctor is not in law entitled to rely on it and exposes himself to possible liability if he does so.

In the context of research on children much obviously turns on what are the relevant legal criteria of competence. Clearly, if a child is competent then its consent must be sought and its refusal respected. If the child is not competent then the doctor must look to someone else.

The law provides some guidance as to the legal competence of children since the Family Law Reform Act 1969, s.8 states that 'the consent of a minor who has attained the age of 16 to any surgical, medical or dental treatment which, in the absence of consent, would constitute a trespass to his person, shall be as effective as it would be if he were of full age; and where a minor has by virtue of this section given an effective consent to any treatment it shall not be necessary to obtain any consent for it from his parent or guardian.' Superficially, this might suggest that 16 is the crucial age: it is for the child to give his consent to medical procedures if he is over 16 and for the parents to give their proxy consent to medical procedures in all cases where the child is under 16. But the situation is not that simple. First, it is not clear whether the section is relevant at all to clinical research for it defines 'surgical, medical or dental treatment' as 'including any procedure undertaken for the purposes of diagnosis, and this section applies to any procedure (including, in particular, the administration of an anaesthetic) which is ancillary to any treatment as it applies to that treatment.' Nothing is said about experimental procedures; and it is strongly arguable that clinical research, at least for non-therapeutic purposes, is not treatment.

Secondly, whatever the section covers, s.8 (3) provides that 'nothing in this section shall be construed as making ineffective any consent which would have been effective if this section had not been enacted.' Thus, the Act throws us back to the Common Law. Clearly, a person who has attained the statutory age of majority, now 18, may consent. Below that age the position, in the absence of judicial authority, is at best obscure. If one can seek guidance from other common law jurisdictions, such as the US and Canada, there are suggestions that a child below the relevant statutory age of majority may still be able to consent to medical procedures in situations of emergency, where speed is essential and parents cannot be traced; and in cases of demonstrated emancipation, for example, where a child has left the family fold and set up an independent home; and where a child is sufficiently mature to understand the nature and consequences of medical procedures and so is able to give an informed consent. The only relevant English decision, however, is that in the case (at present subject to appeal) of *Gillick* v. *West Norfolk AHA* [1985] 1 All ER 533: at first instance Woolf J. held, in the absence of any binding authority, that 'the fact that a child was under 16 did not automatically mean that she could not give any consent to the treatment. Whether a child was capable of giving the necessary consent would depend on the child's maturity and understanding and the nature of the consent required.'

The Court of Appeal, however, rejected this view and decided that until a child reached the 'age of discretion' it was within the custody of its parents and could give no valid consent to medical treatment without parental authority. Any doctor who treated a child without such authority would be behaving unlawfully save in an emergency. The 'age of discretion' was held by the Court to be sixteen in the case of a girl, but fourteen in the case of a boy. It remains to be seen which view of the Common Law the House of Lords will prefer.

Where does this leave the law relating to consent to clinical research? It is clear that a person of 18 or over, who has reached the age of full legal capacity and is not otherwise lacking legal competence, has the capacity to consent to clinical research, provided it is not prohibited by law, whether case law or statute. (Examples exist of conduct which may not be consented to: minors under the age of 18 may not consent to tattooing, by virtue of the Tattooing of Minors Act 1969, and no one may consent to that which the law regards as *malum in se,* for example, that which was designed to maim the person without good reason as justification: see *Att-Gen's Reference (No. 6 of 1980)* [1981] 2 All ER 1057.) It is possible that a child between 16 and 18 also has the legal competence to consent to clinical research if the words 'surgical, medical or dental treatment' in s.8, Family Law Reform Act 1969, are widely construed to include clinical research; or if a child of that age has the maturity and capacity to give an informed consent. With regard to children below 16 the situation is even less clear. Some take the view that such children can never consent to research procedures, whatever the position for medical treatment. Others regard age as not the relevant criterion, but would instead look to the capacity of the child to comprehend the nature and consequences of the procedure proposed. Until this is resolved by Parliament or the courts the cautious lawyer may well be persuaded, *ex abundante cautela,* to opt for the former position, particularly in the light of the Court of Appeals judgment in *Gillick* v. *West Norfolk AHA.*

The view of the law which asserts that the relevant criterion of competence is the ability of the particular individual to comprehend the nature and consequences of the proposed procedure is a standard concerning itself with the intellectual and emotional development of the specific person who is to be subject to research or treatment, and is, therefore, more in keeping with a commitment to respect for the autonomy of each person. It also means that the doctor or researcher involved is under a legal obligation to conduct a careful examination to discover whether a particular child is competent, since questions of comprehension and understanding are not matters which can be answered cursorily or in any routine way.

Even if this view of the law rejects any specific age as determinative of competence, is there not, it is asked, some age below which the law obliges the doctor to assume incompetence. The Medical

Research Council has taken the view that 12 years of age should be the cut-off point; above that, competence would turn on the child's comprehension; below, the child would be incompetent in all circumstances. Of course, to argue in this way is to resurrect the status idea of competence. It is, therefore, better to say, on this view of the law, that it is not concerned with any particular age, but regards progress towards mature judgment as a gradual process.

Obviously, the younger a person is, or the more intrusive the nature of the research, the more difficult it would be to persuade a court that the child had the legal capacity to consent: the law will take due account of relevant psychological expertise concerning the intellectual and emotional development of children in general and the onus on the doctor to demonstrate competence would be heavy. Additionally, in circumstances where a court would be prepared to find that a child had the maturity and understanding to consent to medical treatment, it still might refuse to hold that there was sufficient maturity and understanding to submit to serious, intrusive research procedures. It is instructive to notice the view advanced in the report *Making health care decisions,* prepared in 1982 by the US President's Commission for the Study of Ethical Problems in Medicine and Biomedical and Behavioral Research. The proposal is made that if the child is above 14 years of age then there should be a presumption in favour of competence, which may be displaced by evidence. If, on the other hand, the child is below 14 years old, there would be a presumption against competence, but this would be the starting point for enquiry, rather than obviating the need for further consideration of the particular facts.

Once it is decided that a child is incompetent in law to consent (or refuse to consent) to a procedure, the question becomes, who may consent in its stead. The simple answer is that anyone standing *in loco parentis* to the child may do so. This means that, first the doctor may look to a parent, or, failing that, a legal guardian, or a local authority if the child is in a local authority's care, or seldom, the court, if the child is a ward. Ordinarily of course, it is the parents who must be asked. Where the 'parental rights' are transferred to another body, such as a local authority, that body may technically acquire the 'same powers and duties' as the parent or guardian would have apart from, say, a 'care order' (e.g. Child Care Act 1980, s.10(2)). However, it is likely that its powers and duties *vis à vis* the child may in fact be more restricted than those of a parent: a residual right to be consulted may remain with a parent

(*Re T.* (1963), Ch. 238; see Eekelaar, 'What are parental rights' (1973) 89 LQR 210, 233). One problem which could arise, albeit seldom, is what the doctor is entitled to do when parents disagree with each other. Both parents have equal authority in law to consent on their child's behalf. Good medical practice would counsel in favour of seeking to bring the parents to a common view. If this should not prove possible, the law would appear to be that if the child is ill, in circumstances which could be described as threatening to life or limb, the doctor is entitled to prefer the parent who consents to treatment or therapeutic research over the parent who refuses consent. Where the proposed research is non-therapeutic, whether the child is ill or not, it may be that the doctor should respect the non-consenting parent's view. The reasons are both legal, in that legal advice to the doctor should observe an abundance of caution, when the issue is not clear and the child's health is not at stake, and medical-practical, in that it should be the aim of the doctor to avoid souring any further relationship with the family as a unit whenever possible.

It is important to notice that by recognizing the capacity of a parent or other to consent on behalf of an incompetent child, the law is not abandoning its commitment to respect for autonomy. Indeed, the aim of the law is to maximize the child's opportunity to exercise autonomy in the future. It does so in two ways. First, by regarding as invalid the say-so of the incompetent child, it forbids others from acting on ill-considered choices which would impair the child's ability to come to maturity free from preventable harm. Secondly, it constrains others from consenting on the child's behalf to that which may impair the enjoyment of autonomy at maturity. (See *Re D.* (1976) 1 All ER 326 – a case involving the proposed sterilization of a retarded girl of 11.)

This second point is very important. It makes clear that there are limits to what a parent or other may consent to (or refuse) on behalf of a child. The precise extent of these limits is, again regrettably, not clear, although the Court of Appeal's judgment in *Gillick* v. *West Norfolk AHA* suggests that they are less extensive than previously thought and that the law grants to parents a very considerable degree of decision-making power in relation to their children. Before examining the point in detail, it may be helpful to consider the various legal justifications offered for the conflicting views advanced as to the limits of parental authority. Significantly different answers may be given to questions concerning research on children, depending on which legal justification is advanced, and which of them is most sustainable.

One view, that of 'parents' rights', would have it that a parent has very considerable freedom in making decisions for a child. The most recent and now fashionable development of the argument is that the State's commitment to the family as the basic unit of social life carries with it the implication that the State should respect the authority of the head of the family unit, the parent, and should be slow to interfere in the exercise of parental discretion. Some would say that only a clear and present danger to the health of the child would justify the intervention of the State. Some would go even further and argue that, even in circumstances in which the health of a child were threatened, the parents have a right to choose a course of action which may be idiosyncratic or unorthodox, but which is in keeping with the values embraced by the family. A number of recent cases in the United States have seen this parental right asserted. Clearly, if this view were accepted as the law, the requirement of parental consent in the context of research would potentially be very considerable.

There are a number of weaknesses in this view. The first is that it would have the law subordinate the interests of the child to those of the parent. This tends to go against the tradition of at least twentieth century case law and statute. Take, for example, the cases involving Jehovah's Witnesses when parents have refused their consent to treatment for, or the giving of necessary blood transfusions to, their children. The medical profession's view of the law is that the parent's consent may be dispensed with in such cases, and this view is almost certainly correct. Where applications have been made to courts to remove such children from the legal custody of their parents so that consent can be given by others entrusted with the custody, magistrates' courts have willingly responded.

A parent has no property right over his child which would entitle him to make decisions about the child which, only in undefined but clearly most exceptional circumstances, should be subject to challenge. Such an approach is quite out of line with the development of modern law. (For an interesting analysis, see Eekelaar, 'What are parental rights' (1973) 89 LQR 210.)

The present view of the law is that parents have duties towards their children, the principal one being to safeguard and care for them, and any rights they may have are only such as to enable them to perform these duties. If the analysis begins from the starting point of parental duties, it will be seen that different conclusions about the limits of parental authority may be arrived at.

A second view is captured in the notion of children's rights. This was a view popular in the 1960s and 1970s but is less so at present. It, too, may be said to suffer from certain weaknesses. It resorts again to the self-sustaining assertion of 'rights'. It strikes a balance in familial affairs which can be said to allow parents little discretion or authority, and make them forever subject to the supervision of the State through its various agencies, all of which would be concerned to enquire and ensure that a child's rights were not being threatened or violated by this or that decision.

It would be of great help if a way out of this conflict were available, which would offer a sensible framework for weighing the limits of parental authority. A possible solution, which does no violence to existing law and draws on a legal tradition of great versatility and value, is to speak of the parent as the trustee of the interests of the child. The value of the device would be that it would be one with which the law would be familiar, even though it is used here by way of analogy, since it is not suggested that there is any trust in the strict legal sense of the term. What it would mean is that the parent would be recognized as the person primarily responsible for the affairs of the child. It would mean that the law began with this assumption. It would recognize that in the exercise of that responsibility, the parent would have an appropriate degree of discretion, provided he complies with the terms of the trust, which will be considered below and which, being couched in general language only, would leave him with the ability to exercise discretion based on the special circumstances of each case. It would mean, however, that the parent's authority was limited. It would mean, therefore, that if the terms of the trust were broken, the parent could lose his authority over his child, which would thereafter be exercised by another trustee, e.g. the local authority.

The terms of the trust would then have to be set out. This is what is involved in answering the second question: what may be consented to?

What may be consented to?

The law increasingly is concerned to safeguard a child's interests, and in many areas of family law the welfare of the child is expressed to be the 'first and paramount' consideration. Thus in one case concerning the guardianship of minors, Lord MacDermott said: 'when all the relevant facts, relationship, claims and wishes of parents, risks, choices and other circumstances are taken into account and weighed, the course to be followed will be that which is most in the interests of the child's welfare. This is the first consideration because it is of first importance and paramount because it determines the course to be followed.' Even where the welfare of the child is not the *first* consideration it will still be accorded a high priority when weighed against any competing factors which a court has to take into account (*Richards* v. *Richards* [1983] 2 All ER 807). When the interests and welfare of the child and the public interest in medical research have to be weighed in the balance, what may appear to be only slight differences in approach may well take on considerable significance when determining what, if any, research is legally permissible.

Three criteria are advanced as representing the law on what a parent may consent to on behalf of a child. They are:

(i)   that which is in the best interests of the child;
(ii) that which is in the interests of or redounds to the welfare of the child;
(iii) that which is not against the interests of the child.

Clearly, the first would place the greatest limits on the power of the parent, since it emphasizes that the parent may opt for nothing less than the best. The second criterion is less demanding of the parent or, from another point of view, less protective of the child. More leeway is left to the parent's judgment and no condemnation will follow a decision simply because some think, or events prove, that it was not the best. Perhaps the most important feature of this standard is that the inherent flexibility in the concept of welfare leaves the parent more discretion and casts the burden of proving it on those who argue that any particular course of conduct is not in a child's welfare. The third criterion goes even further. So far from requiring the parent to show that his every act is the best that could be done for the child, he need only show that he has not harmed the child's interests and it is for others to show otherwise. And, merely to show that someone else could have done better, would not, of course, be sufficient.

In the past it has been widely assumed that parents are under the strictest duty; namely, to refrain from consenting to anything which is not in the best interests of the child. Thus, any consent from a parent to non-therapeutic research would be legally invalid and any doctor purporting to act on it would be acting unlawfully. To use the language suggested earlier, it would be a breach of trust by the parent. Particularly influential in causing this view to become the orthodox view in the medical profession were the Report of the Medical Research Council for 1962–3 and the subsequent Department of Health Circular on the 'Supervision of the ethics of clinical research investigations'. The MRC Report stated that, 'in the strict view of the law, parents and guardians of minors cannot give consent on their behalf to any procedures which are of no particular benefit to them and which may carry some risk of harm'. The Departmental Circular advised against inferring that 'the fact that consent has been given by the parent or guardian and that the risk involved is considered negligible will be sufficient to bring such clinical research investigation within the law as it stands'. Such statements were, of course, attempts at educated guesses at what a court would decide. There was not, nor is there, any case law or statute to look to as authority. The MRC Report relied upon the advice of only one distinguished lawyer.

This view of the law has not gone without criticism. It is fair to say that now, in the changed context of attitudes to parental responsibilities and medical research, it is most unlikely that a court would endorse the view taken in 1963 and outlaw non-therapeutic research *in limine*. Instead, it is submitted that a court would adopt as the legal standard the rule that a parent may consent to that which is not against the interests of a child.

Support for this view can be derived from the approach taken to the ordering of blood tests on children to establish paternity. In one case where the Official Solicitor, acting on behalf of a child, objected to submitting the child to blood testing, the House of Lords swept aside the argument that the blood test was not in the best interests of the child in favour of the view that it was not against the child's interests. Lord Reid stated that 'a reasonable parent would have some regard to the general public interest and would not refuse a blood test unless he thought that would clearly be against the interests of the child'. (*S.* v. *S.* [1970] 3 All ER 107,111. This principle is now restated in the Family Law Reform Act 1969, s.21(2).)

Thus, it is submitted that in certain circumstances a parent *is* entitled in law to consent to research investigation on a child.

If the research intervention is intended to be therapeutic, then at face value there seems little difficulty. Clearly, it is not against a child's interests to receive therapy if it is ill. Indeed, such an intervention would satisfy the most demanding criterion of being in the child's best interests. Thus, a parent would in law be entitled to consent to such a research on a child. There is, however, a question which must be considered. Is this view of the law good if there are alternative therapies and one is the subject of research and the other is not? The object of the research in such a case must be either to establish the validity of the therapy under examination, or to compare two available alternative forms of treatment, otherwise the research itself would be unfounded. It now becomes a little less easy to assert that consent to such research is *ex hypothesi* legally valid. If there is an established treatment against which the other is being compared, there may be circumstances when it would be against a child's interests to volunteer it for the research. *A fortiori,* it would not be in the best interests of the child. Where two alternative treatments are being compared there still may be circumstances in which a parent ought not to volunteer a child. To the extent that the researcher must inevitably come to regard the child as both a patient *and* a member of a group subject to research, some would suggest that the doctor's obligation to his patient may not be seen as paramount. Some would then conclude from this that it would be against a child's interests to expose it to such a possibility. It could also be asserted, however, that a keen research doctor might give more detailed attention to his research subjects than to his routine, and possibly less interesting, patients. But it is the nature of the attention rather than the degree which is at issue. If these arguments are taken seriously, and they must be when considering what the law is, or rather what a court would decide if presented with the problem, then some way of solving the problems posed must be found. Otherwise it would appear that, despite the emergence of a less limiting standard of care owed to his child, a parent may still be unsure whether a child may lawfully be volunteered for therapeutic research. The answer, it is submitted, lies in the notion of risk. The parent may consent to a research procedure if, when judged objectively, any risk to which it exposes the child is so small that it would not be against the child's interest to be exposed to it. The benefit to be gained from a research intervention intended to be therapeutic will, by virtue of its being therapeutic, ordinarily outweigh any risks associated with it. Certainly, it would not ordinarily be against a child's interest to be involved in it, and thus the parent would be entitled lawfully to consent to such a research procedure on behalf of a child.

When the proposed research intervention is non-therapeutic the procedure is not, at least prima facie, intended to be in the particular child's interests. But some research procedures in certain circumstances will not be against the interests of the child. Whether the circumstances are appropriate will depend, it is submitted, on the risks to which the child is exposed. So the question becomes, to what risks is it permissible to expose a child in non-therapeutic research? While not outlawing such research altogether, it is submitted that the law will continue to require the parent to observe a high degree of care in protecting a child's interests. Thus, it is submitted that the permissible level of risk allowed by law is low, what some have called minimal risk. The assessment of such risk is, of course, a matter of expert evidence to be assessed in good faith and includes both physical and psychological risk. If it can be shown without argument to be minimal, then the law at present would allow a parent to expose a child to it. This is only another way of saying that allowing a parent intentionally to expose a child to minimal risk will not endanger the child's capacity to mature to autonomy, unharmed by such exposure. And the need to safeguard this capacity must be the criterion of minimal risk.

If this indeed be the law, two questions remain. The first is whether the law ought to be clarified by some appropriate means, despite the fact that it is thought that the views expressed accurately reflect the state of the law. The second is whether some formal procedural mechanism should be introduced to ensure, to the extent possible, that the law, whatever it may be, is observed in practice.

Clarifying the law

It is unlikely that Parliament in the foreseeable future will find time to consider the details of research on children with a view to stating or restating the relevant legal provisions. The alternative method of clarifying the law, by bringing matters before the courts for decision, seems inappropriate. English courts are slow to use their powers to declare what the law is by declaratory judgment, and it would be quite wrong to look to a civil claim for damages, far less a criminal prosecution, as a way of developing a coherent set of principles. It may be, therefore, that another method should be chosen, if the need to clarify the law is thought to be sufficiently strong. This method would involve the preparation of Guidelines or a Code of Practice which would set out the circumstances under which consent to research on children may be given. Such a Code would be drawn up in much the same way as the existing Codes on, for example, organ donation for the purposes of transplant, or the determination of brain-stem death. Although not having the force of law, such a Code would have a very strong persuasive effect, representing as it would the product of considered deliberation, in the context of an uncertain and potentially flexible legal regime, by a group representative of all appropriate constituencies. As with existing Codes, compliance with its provision by the doctor or researcher would be prima facie evidence that he had acted lawfully. The onus would be on others then to show that the Code was wrong in law. Given the circumstances of its creation, it would be doubtful if any court would so decide. Furthermore, any doctor or researcher who did not observe the provisions of the Code would prima facie risk being deemed to have acted unlawfully and would have the burden of demonstrating otherwise.

Of course, if recourse to such a Code is thought still to leave matters too much in doubt, then Parliamentary action is the only available alternative and an appropriately drafted Bill would have to be prepared.

Ensuring compliance with the law

It is, of course, one thing to have a statement of what the law requires and another to ensure that the law is in fact observed. To suggest that some sort of formal mechanism be contemplated so as to ensure that the law is observed is not, of course, to impugn the integrity of doctors and researchers or of parents. Rather it is to suggest that, where there exists a standard which gives parents considerable discretion as to what they may consent to on behalf of a child, some check may be appropriate to ensure that a particular exercise of discretion is not against a particular child's interests, whether because of enthusiasm for the project, desire to participate or be seen to help, or just poor judgment. For this reason a proposal has been made that a child's advocate or guardian of the child's interests be involved before consent is given to involve a child in research. Perhaps, the best term to describe such a person is 'the child's friend'. This would capture the idea that his role is to speak for the child and to weigh all proposals in terms of the effect they may have, physically or psychologically, on the child. (Similar provisions have recently been introduced in to the mental health legislation (Mental Health Act 1983, ss.56–64).)

Those who call for the interposition of such a person between the parent and the researcher see him as having obviously a greater role in the context of non-therapeutic research intervention. The advantages of formalizing the appointment of such a person are several. First, ethics committees would be reminded of their obligation to consider the interests of children in research by the knowledge that the child's advocate or friend would be involved in any particular decisions to be made. Secondly, doctors, researchers, and parents, each time a child is considered as the possible subject of a research, would have to defend rationally the choice of this child and the validity of the exercise. This is not to say that they do not do so now, but rather that requiring them to do so to others can only enhance the protection of the child's interests. Thirdly, the existence of formal legal criteria for research interventions coupled with a procedure for ensuring compliance with them will serve to reassure the public and thereby create a climate in which appropriate research can be conducted in a climate of understanding and shared endeavour.

Despite these arguments a majority of the working group decided against recommending the introduction of a child advocate scheme. Instead, the majority favoured encouraging each ethics committee to ensure that its membership was such that it was capable of taking particular account of the interests of any children considered for research.

Addendum in proof: The House of Lords, by a majority, reversed the Court of Appeal's decision in the *Gillick* case. Lord Scarman said 'the parental right to determine whether or not their minor child below the age of 16 will have medical treatment terminates *if and when the child achieves a sufficient understanding and intelligence to enable him or her to understand fully what is proposed*'. This ruling may extend to consent to research and not be limited to treatment.

7

Can children permit research?

The previous chapter has discussed the legal constraints on clinical research, and, in particular, the legal requirements for consent to research. It has been seen that there are few specific rules to guide a researcher, and that the best advice remains that of Edmund Burke: 'It is not what a lawyer tells me I may do; but what humanity, reason and justice tell me I ought to do.'

There is, however, one aspect of research on children for which humanity and reason may not readily provide an answer: it concerns the age at which a child may permit a research procedure on himself, if indeed there is such an age before that of his legal majority. Since consent is usually taken to mean the legally significant permission given by a parent or guardian, the word 'assent' is commonly used to denote a child's permission for the performance of a research procedure on himself. There is considerable variation in the ages at which different researchers request a child's assent to a research procedure. In the study by Janofsky and Starfield[1] of researchers' perceptions of risk, referred to in Chapter 5, they sought information also about the criteria used to decide whether a child was capable of giving assent. Three-quarters of the respondents said that the researcher used his clinical judgement to assess the maturity of the child. Most of the other respondents 'indicated that the child's chronologic age was the sole criterion used to gauge maturity', and the ages of 5, 7, 9, 10, 12, 13, and 15 years were given by various respondents as the minimum age for seeking assent. The survey of research ethics committees reported in Chapter 8 showed that only 10 per cent of such committees in England and Wales specify an age from which the assent of a child must be sought: the commonest age specified was 16 years, the range being from 10 years to 17 years. The Medical Research Council in its 1963 statement[2] suggested that English courts would not consider a child of less than 12 years as capable of giving such assent, and that Scottish courts would take 14 years as the minimum.

That there should be such a variety in the suggested ages of assent may in part be explained by the considerable and obvious differences in the rate of development of different children. Some children may never develop to a stage at which they are capable of mature moral reasoning, while a recent English television programme on the ethics of genetic engineering showed the 8- and 10-year-old sons of a moral philosopher to be quite capable of forming mature judgements. Most children, however, develop their capacities for moral judgement in a relatively uniform manner, and the results of a few relevant studies allow one to suggest that there need not be such a great variety in the age from which assent is sought.

Theories of child development

The first, but rather indirect, evidence that might be considered comes from the studies of cognitive and moral development by Piaget, and their later elaboration by Kohlberg, in particular. Piaget started his examination of how children develop a respect for moral rules by examining the effects of rules in the games that they played.[3] Up to the age of 5 or 6 years, he found that children tend to play games egocentrically with little concern for others around them. By the age of 7 or 8 years, however, they had a strongly developed sense of shared rules, so that they could play together, while expecting everyone to stick firmly to the rules. At that age a child believed that the rules had been provided by adults, and so he was at a stage of moral realism, believing that moral rules had an existence independent of himself. It was at a later stage, around the age of 10 or 11 years, that co-operative play had developed to the point at which rules could be altered by the consent of the players, and were no longer absolute rules imposed from outside. Moral subjectivism had replaced moral realism.

Kohlberg extended this scheme by examining the responses of children to a set of hypothetical moral dilemmas that he had developed. He suggested three levels of the development of moral judgement – pre-conventional, conventional, and post-conventional – in which 'conventional' referred to conventional conformity to rules.[4] In the pre-conventional stage, the prime motive was the avoidance of punishment or the obtaining of rewards. In the conventional stage, the need to be a good person both in one's own opinion and that of others, some sort of belief in the Golden Rule, and a desire to support authority, provided much of the motive. In the post-conventional stage, there was 'an implicit notion of a contract with others and a democratically accepted set of laws, and this was followed by a morality of self-determined individual principles of conscience which could transcend such laws.'[5] It is difficult to supply specific ages at which the three levels of development of moral judgement, according to Kohlberg, develop; in certain circumstances, moreover, pre-conventional behaviour may persist for some time after conventional behaviour has developed, and post-conventional behaviour may never develop. In general, however, 7- or 8-year-olds display pre-conventional behaviour. Early parts of conventional behaviour – such as living up to one's parents' expectations – develop in pre-adolescents of perhaps 10 or 11 years old. A later part of conventional behaviour is the development of the ability to look beyond the point-of-view of one's own close group in order to see one's behaviour from the perspective of society as a whole: such a development tends to start in mid-adolescence, from the age of about 14 years. Post-conventional behaviour, when it develops, generally does so from the age of 18 upwards.

These two theories have been subject to a variety of criticisms. The main problem for the present study is that they do not greatly assist a researcher wondering about the need for assent. There are perhaps a few generalizations that might be made. It seems likely that a fully informed consent, in which a prospective research subject has taken full account of the implications of a project for society as well as for himself, is only possible when the later stages of conventional moral judgement have been reached. In some instances, it may be that such consent requires a post-conventional level of moral reasoning. At an earlier stage of development, it is unlikely that a child with purely pre-conventional moral judgement will have any concept of the implications for others of his involvement as a research subject. But as soon as some elements of conventional moral judgement develop, some simple ideas of performing acts now for the benefit of others at a later date will be present. This is not, of course, to deny that altruistic impulses may be observed in much younger children, when another person may receive an immediate benefit. Since early conventional moral judgement may develop by the age of 10, some of the criteria for seeking assent may be present from that age upwards.

Some practical studies

Various studies may help to elaborate the above ideas. The study by Schwartz of 'Children's concepts of research hospitalization'[6] was considered earlier in the context of emotional risks to children when taking part in research. In that example the research programme was a relatively complicated study of human growth hormone deficiency and supplementation; before entry into the study, children had several opportunities to discuss it and to find out what would happen to them. Yet, when interviewed during the study, none of the children aged 11 years or under showed any awareness that their stay in hospital had anything to do with research.

Schwartz's findings may be contrasted with those of Lewis *et al.* during a rather simpler study.[7] During the Swine Flu Affair in the United States in 1976, the children in an elementary school in Los Angeles were approached to become subjects in a trial of the swine-flu vaccine. The authors went to the classrooms of the 6- to 9-year-old children, described the nature of the study to them in outline, and invited questions. The question session was non-directive, but, even so, all except the 6-year-old children succeeded in eliciting from the authors all the information regarding swine flu itself, and the risks and benefits of the vaccination, that the authors considered necessary for informed consent. Having done so, 46 per cent of the children then declined to participate. The remainder either agreed or were uncertain: their parents were asked for consent and 15 per cent gave it. That nearly half the children declined to take part suggests that there was no group pressure to do so. But the study does not provide any evidence about the individual child's ability or competence to form a judgement: it merely shows that in a group setting children as young as 7 years old may be able to elicit the necessary information about a relatively simple research procedure to make a decision whether or not to participate.

The study of Lewis *et al.* produced a response from Kegeles and Lund[8] that was perhaps a little wide of the mark, but contained one interesting suggestion. That was the assertion that such a low rate of volunteering was alarming since it might encourage other workers to bypass the children and to go directly to the parents to ask for consent. They reported their own experience of asking seventh

grade children (aged 11 to 13 years) to volunteer for caries prevention studies, involving either three topical fluoride applications or
the use of a fluoridated mouth rinse daily at home. In most cases
the volunteering rate had been 95–100 per cent, and it was always
greater than 90 per cent. It is important to note, however, that they
were using older children, in Kohlberg's conventional stage, and
were asking for volunteers for a relatively painless procedure.

Children's knowledge of health and illness

Several studies recently have looked at the understanding that
children or adolescents have about health and illness. Perrin and
Gerrity,[9] for example, used an interviewing technique with open-
ended questions in a group of 128 children varying from kindergarten level to eighth grade, i.e. from age 5½ on average, to age 13
years. Kindergarten children understand illness either in terms of
magic, or as the result of their breaking some rule. At age 9 years,
'children believe all illness to be caused by germs whose very
presence is sufficient to make a child sick'. It is only at the age of 12
or 13 years that children start to have an understanding of the multiple causes of illness. In their conclusion, Perrin and Gerrity
suggest that adults frequently assume that children have a more
sophisticated understanding of illness than appears to be the case;
they also indicate some evidence that children in hospital have less
advanced ideas of the cause of illness than healthy children not in
hospital. A study of adolescents aged 11 to 15 by Millstein *et al.*[10]
showed that their conceptions of illness were closer to those of
children than to those of adults.

Other studies of children's conceptions of health and illness
serve to show the difficulties in obtaining comparable results from
different groups of children. Kister and Patterson, for instance,
examined the ideas about causes of illness held by healthy children
aged between 4½ years and 9½ years.[11] They looked first at the
idea of contagion, asking the children whether ailments such as a
cold, toothache, or a scraped knee could be caught from another
child. By the age of 7½, children rarely called contagious an
ailment that was not. They also examined the 'use of immanent
justice' as an explanation for illness: i.e. they tried to find out the
extent to which the children regarded illness as a punishment. Few
of the oldest group — average age 9½ years – regarded illness as a
punishment, but most of the younger children did. These results

suggest that children may develop some understanding of the causes of illness at a younger age than was suggested by Perrin and Gerrity.[9]

In the United Kingdom, Eiser and colleagues have asked school children about the inside of their bodies,[12] and about their knowledge of health and illness.[13] They were surprised at how little the children, aged 6 to 12 years, knew about their bodies, both in absolute terms and in comparison with the levels of knowledge reported in American studies. Thus, 6-year-olds were able to mention only three internal organs, the most common being the heart, blood, and bones, while 12-year-olds mentioned seven organs on average. The functions of various body parts were examined by asking the children which parts were involved in processes such as eating, breathing, getting rid of waste and swimming. Eiser and Patterson[12] concluded: 'For the 6-year-olds it is apparent that food enters the stomach but they are unclear as to what then happens. The interconnection between the digestive and excretory systems begins to emerge among the 8-year-olds, but any further connections with the circulatory system are not made even among the 12-year-olds.' Three out of twenty-six 12-year-olds did not mention the lungs as being involved with breathing, and five of them could not answer the question about getting rid of waste at all; fourteen – just over half – were able to mention the brain as being involved in controlling limb movements for swimming.

Eiser *et al.*[13] asked a different group of children, aged 6 to 11 years, to define 'being healthy', what they must do to stay healthy, and what they knew about ailments such as chickenpox, nits in the hair, and cancer. The children tended to define being healthy in terms of eating a good diet and taking exercise. Most of the 6-year-olds could not think of any way of preventing illness, but from the age of 8 years upwards, almost all the children could do so. Interestingly, 55 per cent of the 6-year-olds did not know what an injection was, while only 5 per cent of the 8-year-olds did not know. In general, the level of knowledge about diseases and their prevention was thought to be poor, as perhaps exemplified by whooping-cough, about which only a quarter even of the 12-year-olds knew anything. These two papers suggest that a certain amount of understanding about health and illness develops particularly between the ages of 6 and 8 years, but that considerable areas of ignorance remain even by 12 years of age.

The studies of Perrin and Gerrity,[9] Kister and Patterson,[11] and

Eiser and colleagues [12,13] are concerned primarily with matters of fact – the knowledge that children of various ages have about health and illness. Such knowledge is likely to be considerably influenced by the social and educational backgrounds of the children concerned; it does not, of itself, bear any relation to the capacity of the same children to form mature judgements. The ability to make competent decisions about medical treatment or participation in clinical research depends on an understanding of relevant facts, however, and it is therefore important for investigators to be aware of how little knowledge of health and illness many children may have. Information about the abilities of children to form mature judgements must be sought elsewhere.

Competence to consent or assent

Probably the most directly relevant information about the ability of children to provide assent comes from a study by Weithorn.[14] She studied a total of 96 children to examine developmental differences in their competence to make informed treatment decisions. Competence is introduced as a legal concept, being required, with 'information' and 'voluntariness', for legal validation of a patient's consent to treatment. Legal commentators have identified tests of competence as:

(a) evidence of a choice being made by the patient;
(b) a 'reasonable' outcome for that choice;
(c) evidence of 'rational' thought in making the choice;
(d) comprehension of the risks, benefits, and alternatives.

The last category can be divided into 'factual understanding' and an appreciation of the implications of the variables presented.

Formal operational thought is needed to be able to carry out (a) to (d): Piaget suggests that such thought starts at about age 11 and is well developed by age 14. Thus, one group of 24 subjects was 9 years old, and another 14 years old, with two groups of college students aged 18 and 21 years as adult 'controls'. All subjects were white and spoke English only. Hypothetical treatment dilemmas were presented to the subjects; since the latter were all healthy, it was felt that there would be a better comparison between the groups. The dilemmas had a range of complexity (i.e. number of options), content (i.e. types of health problems) and difficulty (i.e.

the degree to which the reasonable options were clearcut rather than ambiguous).

Twenty-five dilemmas were pilot-tested, and four, describing problems in diabetes, epilepsy, depression, and enuresis, were chosen. Information given included the nature of the problem, alternative treatments and their expected benefits, possible risks and side-effects, and the consequences of failure to treat; descriptions used vocabulary appropriate to the age of the subjects. An interview schedule was developed concentrating on the four tests of competence. A panel of 20 'experts' scored the 'reasonableness' of the treatment options in the dilemmas presented and the mean score for any option became the score given to a subject who chose that option (1 = completely unreasonable, 5 = completely reasonable). Subjects also scored a point on a separate 'Scale of rational reasons' for each of several responses to questions about what they had taken into account when deciding on a treatment option. The final scale measured subjects' understanding and was divided into 'Rote recall' and 'Inference', which examined the subjects' understanding of the information disclosed in the dilemma and their ability to make inferences about that information. The groups (12 males and 12 females at each age level) were found to be comparable in terms of verbal intelligence and social position (mean IQ approx 120; middle-class). The procedure took 2 to 2½ hours.

Weithorn found the following results:

(a) *Reasonable outcome:* the only significant difference in this category involved the depression dilemma, in which a choice was given between in-patient, out-patient, or no treatment. In-patient treatment was selected by 50 per cent of the 9-year-olds, 17 per cent of the 14-year-olds, 8 per cent of the 18-year-olds, and none of the 21-year-olds.

(b) *Rational reasons:* for each dilemma the 9-year-olds scored significantly lower than each of the other three groups. Overall, there was no difference between the 14-year-olds and the two adult groups, although on one dilemma the 14-year-olds scored just significantly lower.

(c) *Scale of understanding:* Again, the 9-year-olds scored significantly lower than the other three age groups, but the 14-year-olds produced scores almost identical to those of the adult group.

The conclusions drawn were, first, that on all tests of competence the 14-year-olds demonstrated levels of competence as great as that of the two adult groups; secondly, that according to standards of reasonable outcome, the 9-year-olds were as competent as adults, although on measures of understanding and rationality they scored significantly lower. In fact, when questioned afterwards about what they had taken into account when making their decisions, the 9-year-olds overwhelmingly identified one or two of the most salient factors, while failing to consider more complex or multiple factors. The experiments were, however, done on intelligent, white, middle-class, healthy North American children, and so may not be generalizable.

The competence of legal minors has also been examined in the United States in relation to what are known as 'Miranda' rights. *Miranda* v. *Arizona*[15] was a legal case which established that anyone accused of a crime must be informed both of his right to legal assistance and his right to remain silent so as not to incriminate himself. Information obtained by the police subsequently can only be used as evidence in court if the accused gave a 'knowing, intelligent and voluntary' waiver of his rights. A later case in the US Supreme Court extended the right to legal minors.[16] Grisso and his colleagues have studied both juveniles and adults in various detention centres in order to evaluate their understanding of the standard warnings given to accused persons about their rights to silence and legal assistance.[17] He summarized his conclusions as follows:[18]

(a) the vast majority of juveniles aged 14 years and younger do not comprehend the meaning of the *Miranda* warnings and their implications sufficiently to provide a meaningful waiver of their rights;

(b) 15- and 16-year-olds demonstrated comprehension not significantly different from that of adults, unless their IQ was 80 or less;

(c) at least a quarter of adults failed to show a legally adequate understanding of the *Miranda* warnings;

(d) comprehension of their rights by juveniles was not related to race, socioeconomic status or previous experience with the police or courts.

In an earlier review, Grisso had also examined the ability of minors to consent to treatment.[19] He concluded that there was no case for allowing independent consent by those under 11 years old, and that conversely there was no psychological evidence to support the customary legal refusal to accept that consent provided by minors of 15 years and upwards was competent. He regarded the ages 11–14 as a transitional period, in which some individuals might give a competent consent, but during which it was necessary to make allowance for the deference to authority generally shown by minors of that age. Such deference may well continue to a later age, when a minor would otherwise be considered competent, as shown in a study by Lewis.[20] She compared the ways in which minors and adults came to decisions to terminate pregnancies. The minors in her study, aged 13 to 17 years, were significantly more likely than the adults to regard their decisions as having been 'externally' determined, generally by means of parental pressure, whether or not the parents actually knew of the pregnancy.

The evidence of the various sources reviewed above not surprisingly fails to provide any specific ages at which one might prescribe that assent either must or must not be solicited from the child research subject. It does, however, suggest that there are two ages which represent significant turning points for children with the average developmental levels of those ages. At about the age of 7, the knowledge of children about health and illness reaches a level at which it becomes possible to communicate with them about such matters. They are also likely to be in a later pre-conventional stage of the development of moral judgement, in which there is the beginning of the recognition of the interests of others. This stage of development has long been recognized by the Roman Catholic church which has traditionally held that moral responsibility begins at the age of 7.

The second significant turning point comes at about the age of 14 years, when both the observations of Piaget and Kohlberg, and the more directed studies of, for instance, Weithorn suggest that a minor has achieved a level of competence in making decisions that differs from that of an adult only in terms of less experience and information and not in terms of ability to make a judgement. This turning-point has been specifically recognized in the field of medical treatment and research by one legislature. The South African Anatomical Donations and Post-Mortem Examinations Act 1970, says that a child over the age of 14, who is capable of validly expressing his will, can consent to the removal for 'any therapeutic or scientific purpose of blood, skin or other tissue which is replaceable by natural processes of repair' from his body, without parental consent.[21]

In the United Kingdom, neither statute nor case law gives any direct support to 14 years being the age at which children are competent to give consent to medical treatment or research. But a recent House of Lords decision[22] alludes in passing to 14 years being the age of competence to consent in another context. The case concerned the snatching by a father of his minor child who was a ward of court in the care and control of her mother. It was decided that it was possible for a parent to be convicted of kidnapping his minor child, and that the absence of consent by the child to being taken away was a material ingredient of the offence. In his judgement, Lord Brandon stated: 'In the case of a very young child, it would not have the understanding or the intelligence to give its consent, so that absence of consent would be a necessary inference from its age. In the case of an older child, however, it must, I think, be a question of fact for a jury whether the child concerned has sufficient understanding and intelligence to give its consent; if, but only if, the jury considers that a child has these qualities, it must then go on to consider whether it has been proved that the child did not give its consent. While the matter will always be for the jury alone to decide, I should not expect a jury to find at all frequently that a child under 14 had sufficient understanding and intelligence to give its consent.'

Conclusions

Before the age of 7 years (by which is meant the developmental age of an average 7-year-old, rather than a precise chronological age that would apply to all children equally) attempts to obtain a child's assent (by which is meant a permission given by the child that does not, however, have the legal force of consent) are likely to be meaningless, and it is more important simply to tell the child, as much as possible using his level of language, what is going to be done. From the age of 7 years upwards, it becomes important that an investigator should try to obtain the assent of a child subject.

The nearer the child is to 14 years old, the more important does his assent to a research procedure become. Nevertheless, in the age range 7 to 14 years, he will not usually have reached an adult level of moral judgement, and it would not be improper in some circumstances for his refusal of assent to be overridden. In particular, it seems reasonable that the consent of a parent or guardian should override the refusal of assent of a 7- to 14-year-old to a therapeutic research procedure. On the other hand, if the research procedure is not intended to benefit the child and is therefore non-therapeutic, it should not in general be carried out if the child refuses assent. From the age of 14 years upwards it appears that children, although legally minors, are as competent as adults to decide and their views should therefore be given as much consideration as those of the parents. It is suggested that from the age of 14 years upwards, the adolescent subject's refusal to give consent, whether to therapeutic or non-therapeutic research procedures, should be binding. If the adolescent consents to participate in research, then the parents' or guardian's refusal of consent should probably only be binding in the case of non-therapeutic research. The adolescent should in general be able to take part in therapeutic research, if he so consents; the more the research procedure would appear to be in the child's interest, the less weight the parent's refusal should have. Such consent, given by an adolescent, should be recorded in writing, although usually a child's assent need only be oral.

References

1. Janofsky, J. and Starfield, B. Assessment of risk in research on children. *J. Pediat.* **98**, 842–6 (1981).
2. Medical Research Council. Responsibility in investigations on human subjects. In *Report of the Medical Research Council for the year 1962–63*, pp.21–25. HMSO, London (1964).
3. Piaget, J. *The moral judgement of the child* (translated by M. Gabain). Routledge & Kegan Paul, London (1932).
4. Kohlberg, L. Moral stages and moralization: the cognitive-developmental approach. In *Moral development and Behavior: theory, research and social issues* (ed. T. Lickona). Holt, Rinehart, & Winston, New York (1976).
5. Graham, P. J. Moral development. In *Scientific foundations of developmental psychiatry* (ed. M. Rutter) pp.339–53. Heinemann, London (1980).
6. Schwartz, A. H. Children's concepts of research hospitalization. *New Engl. J. Med.* **287**, 589–92 (1972).

7. Lewis, C. E., Lewis, M. A., and Ifekwunigue, M. Informed consent by children and participation in an influenza vaccine trial. *Am. J. Public Hlth* **68**, 1079–82 (1978).
8. Kegeles, S. S. and Lund, A. K. Informed consent of children in field trials (letter). *Am. J. Public Hlth* **69**, 722 (1979).
9. Perrin, E. C. and Gerrity, P. S. There's a demon in your belly: children's understanding of illness. *Pediatrics* **67**, 841–9 (1981).
10. Millstein, S. G., Adler, N. E., and Irwin, C. E. Conceptions of illness in young adolescents. *Pediatrics* **68**, 834–9 (1981).
11. Kister, M. C. and Patterson, C. J. Children's conceptions of the causes of illness: Understanding of contagion and use of immanent justice. *Child Development* **51**, 839–46 (1980).
12. Eiser, C. and Patterson, D. 'Slugs and snails and puppy-dog tails' – children's ideas about the inside of their bodies. *Child: care, health and development* **9**, 233–40 (1983).
13. ——, ——, and Eiser, J. R. Children's knowledge of health and illness: implications for health education. *Child: care, health and development* **9**, 285–92 (1983).
14. Weithorn, L. A. and Campbell, S. B. The competency of children and adolescents to make informed treatment decisions. *Child Development* **53**, 1589–98 (1982).
15. *Miranda* v. *Arizona*, 348 US 436 (1966).
16. *In re Gault*, 387 US 1 (1967).
17. Grisso, T. *Juveniles' waiver of rights: legal and psychological competence.* Plenum, New York (1981).
18. Grisso, T. Juveniles' consent in delinquency proceedings. In *Children's competence to consent* (eds G. B. Melton, G. P. Koocher, and M. J. Saks) pp.131–48. Plenum, New York (1983).
19. —— and Vierling, L. Minors' consent to treatment: a developmental perspective. *Professional Psychology* **9**, 412–27 (1978).
20. Lewis, C. C. A comparison of minors' and adults' pregnancy decisions. *Am. J. Orthopsychiatry* **50**, 446–53 (1980).
21. Burchell, J. M. Non-therapeutic medical research on children. *S. African Law J.* **95**, 193–216 (1978).
22. *R.* v. *D. All England Law Reports* **2**, 449–58 (1984).

8

Research ethics committees

As one views the considerable literature available discussing the ethical review of clinical research on human beings, it is hard to believe that only twenty years ago procedures for such review were generally non-existent. The problem with most of the writings in this field is that they are highly repetitive statements of opinion; only seldom does one find any hard data about the actual structure and methods of working of the committees that have been established to provide ethical review. The working group found, in particular, that no information was available about the ways in which British research ethics committees examined proposals for research on children. It therefore decided to undertake a survey to try to fill some of this gap: the results of the survey are reported in this chapter. First, however, it is worth examining further some of the history of the ethical review of clinical research that was touched on in the Introduction.

Early development of ethical review

It has sometimes been suggested [1] that Thomas Percival in his *Medical ethics*,[2] published in 1803, was the first to argue that a doctor proposing to undertake research should submit to peer review of his project before starting. This interpretation does, however, seem to read rather too much into his works. Percival was a respected physician to the Manchester Infirmary, whose main purpose in *Medical ethics* was to establish a code of good conduct for physicians and surgeons. He was concerned in particular to produce 'harmonious intercourse' among the 'gentlemen of the Faculty' – i.e. those doctors working in the hospital – which would 'naturally produce frequent consultations'. He expected such consultations between doctors for routine cases, and stated that 'no important operation should be determined upon, without ,a consultation of the Physicians and Surgeons'. It is hardly surprising, therefore, that when he supported the trial of 'new remedies and new methods of chirurgical treatment', he also stated that 'no such trials should be instituted without a previous consultation of the Physicians or Surgeons, according to the nature of the case'. The consultation was for him a routine part of medical etiquette; the use of a new treatment would have been innovative therapy rather than research because it would have been most unlikely to have been carried out in a systematic way. An example of the difference in medical practice nearly two centuries ago is that when he discussed 'venesection', he was thinking, not of taking a blood sample in order to make measurements on it, but of blood-letting for the sake, supposedly, of therapy.

The first modern guidelines for the conduct of clinical research were produced by the German Ministry of the Interior in 1931;[3] they have been discussed in the Introduction. They were produced in response to frequent allegations, in both the German Press and Parliament, of unethical conduct by doctors during the previous decade. At that time Germany had a thriving chemical industry, collaboration with which had enabled researchers to develop the first chemotherapeutic agents for infections such as malaria, trypanosomiasis, and leishmaniasis, and led to animal trials of Prontosil, the first sulphonamide, in 1933. Howard-Jones[4] suggests that doctors may well not have been 'sufficiently critical in exploiting the multiplicity of new remedies' placed at their disposal. In the midst of the public debate, the Berlin Medical Board suggested that there should be an official body to regulate all proposed experiments on humans: it seems likely that this was the first time that peer review of modern clinical research had been suggested. Little came of the suggestion, however. There is no mention of the need for peer review or for ethical review in the 1931 German guidelines,[3] in the 1947 Nuremberg Code,[5] or in the original, 1964, version of the Helsinki Declaration.[6] The 1963 Medical Research Council statement[7] does not suggest that ethical review be made a formal procedure, but does suggest that heads of research departments, specialized learned societies, and the editors of journals all have a responsibility, with individual investigators, to ensure the maintenance of appropriate ethical standards.

The first formal requirement for ethical review was that made in

1966 by the Surgeon-General of the United States Public Health Service;[8] before any grant could be made by the Public Health Service in support of research on human beings, that research should have been reviewed by a committee of the researcher's institutional associates to determine the rights and welfare of the subjects, the appropriateness of the methods to be used to gain informed consent, and the risks and potential benefits of the research. Since 1966 a variety of further rules and laws have been made in the United States of America to regulate the ethical review of clinical research, including, in particular, the National Research Act of 1974.[9] All federally-funded clinical research has to be reviewed by a previously approved 'Institutional Review Board'; various rules limit the permissible structure and functions of IRBs. The rules do not, however, apply to research that is not funded by some branch of the US Government, although considerable debate continues as to whether IRBs in institutions in which some research is federally-funded should be required to review all research in such institutions.[10]

When the first formal rules for ethical review were made by the US Surgeon-General in 1966, there were some committees already in existence that had been established to provide peer review of research on humans. In 1960, Welt[11] sent a questionnaire to approximately 80 university departments of medicine in the US; 66 replied, of which 24 either already had, or were in favour of having, a committee to review problems in human experimentation. In 1962, the Law-Medicine Research Institute of Boston University followed up Welt's survey. Fifty-two out of 86 departments of medicine replied, 22 of which reported 'that they had review committees that examined questions concerning the use of human subjects'.[8] The sort of questions examined, however, were 'such matters as general research design, qualifications of the investigator, safety of the subject, and financial support of the study'. These committees did not necessarily, therefore, provide adequate ethical review of research on humans, a finding confirmed by Barber in his national survey,[12] when he found that 38 per cent of committees existing before the 1966 US Public Health Service regulations had to improve their procedures in order to satisfy the regulations.

The first mention of ethical review committees in the United Kingdom appears to be in the letter to the President of the Royal College of Physicians that led to that College setting up its committee on the supervision of the ethics of clinical research investigations in institutions.[13] The letter stated that one or more ethical review committees were being established in institutions in the United Kingdom that received grants from the US Public Health Service, in order to satisfy the latter's 1966 regulations. The College committee advised, in 1967, that a group of doctors 'should satisfy itself of the ethics of all proposed investigations' in medical institutions.

In the same year, the idea of having a non-medical member of such a committee was raised for the first time in the United Kingdom by Pappworth in his book *Human guinea pigs*.[14] He suggested that the lay member should, for preference, be a lawyer. A study carried out by the US National Institutes of Health in 1968 of 142 IRBs showed that only 27 per cent were not limited in membership to immediate peer groups of the researchers, but included members of other professions or lay people. In 1969 the US Public Health Service altered its regulations to require lay membership of institutional review boards. The 1973 revision of the Royal College of Physicians' report also suggested that there should be a lay member of research ethics committees in the United Kingdom. The 1975 revision of the Declaration of Helsinki did not, however, make any such suggestion, and in fact the only possible suggestion of ethical review contained in it is section 1.2: 'The design and performance of each experimental procedure involving human subjects should be clearly formulated in an experimental protocol which should be transmitted to a specially appointed independent committee for consideration, comment and guidance.' It is only in the 1982 *Proposed international guidelines for biomedical research involving human subjects*[15] that ethical review committees are more fully discussed, and the statement made that 'the membership may include . . . laymen qualified to represent community, cultural and moral values'.

It is evident therefore that the requirement of ethical review of proposed research on human subjects is of relatively recent origin. The purposes of such review have been summarised by Levine[1] as that:

1. There should be informed consent.
2. There should be good research design.
3. There should be competent investigators.
4. There should be a favourable balance of harms and benefits.
5. There should be equitable selection of subjects.

6. There should be compensation for research-induced injury.

It is inevitable, however, that such a relatively new procedure will result in different committees having widely varying ideas of the importance of each of the above purposes, and very different methods of trying to achieve them. The need for lay membership of ethical review committees, for instance, having been suggested for the first time only eighteen years ago, is by no means universally accepted. It is accepted in the United States because it is the law that institutional review boards reviewing federally funded research must have a lay member.[16] While there are a few countries that have embodied rules about research on humans in their health laws, it is only in the United States that there is a comprehensive set of laws and regulations for the protection of human research subjects. Information is, however, available about the process of ethical review in a number of countries: Argentina,[17] Australia,[18] Canada,[19,20] Chile,[21] Denmark,[22] Finland,[22] France,[23] India,[24,25] Korea,[26] Malaysia,[27] Mexico,[28] New Zealand,[29] Nigeria,[30] Norway,[22] Philippines,[31] Sweden,[32,33] United Kingdom (see next paragraph), and the United States of America.[34–36] Fluss[37] has reviewed the requirements for the proper conduct of research on humans as specified in the laws and national codes of medical ethics of approximately thirty countries. Several of these countries have semi-official systems in which there is strong pressure, but no legal requirement, to seek ethical review. The strong pressure is often exerted by funding bodies that will only consider proposals that have been accepted by an ethical review committee.

Ethical review in the United Kingdom

Since 1966, ethical review of proposed clinical research in the United Kingdom has been undertaken by research ethics committees, the number of which has gradually increased. The two reports of the Royal College of Physicians each gave impetus to the establishment of such committees, and this was reinforced by the Department of Health and Social Security's circular in 1975,[38] which was however advisory in nature. There have been various studies of the structure and of aspects of the functioning of single committees or groups of committees. One study examined all the known committees in Scotland,[39] deriving information about their size and composition in terms of doctors, nurses, and lay people, their interpretations of their function, the methods by which they worked, ethical problems that they had encountered, and their own assessment of their effectiveness. Another survey[40] was undertaken of committees in health districts where there is a teaching hospital: this examined the size and composition of the committees, the number of projects considered, and the application forms used. Other reports have looked in greater depth at the work of individual committees. Two of these committees served a teaching hospital (Southampton[41] and University College Hospital in London),[42] one served a district (Harrow) that includes the Clinical Research Centre at Northwick Park Hospital,[43] and two served areas before the 1982 reorganization, one being a 'teaching area' (Newcastle),[44] and the other (Durham)[45] being 'non-teaching area'. Only the report of the Harrow District Ethical Committee mentions that the particular problems of undertaking research on children had been discussed by the committee: it approves the use of the risk/benefit ratio in assessing such research, and quotes a legal opinion that a parent may give a legally effective consent to non-therapeutic procedures on a child.

In the absence of more specific information about the ways in which research ethics committees examine proposals for research on children, this working group decided to undertake a survey of such committees, in order to be able to take into account current practice, when making its recommendations. While it was realized that the types of information that can be obtained by the use of a questionnaire are necessarily limited, the time and money to undertake a substantial survey by interviewing chairmen and members of research ethics committees were not available. A questionnaire was therefore designed which would examine principally the composition of committees, their working procedures, the outcome of proposals considered for research on children, and the procedures that they required for obtaining consent to research on children. The questionnaire in full is contained in Appendix A.

Survey of research ethics committees

Committees and respondents

Since research ethics committees in Scotland had already been surveyed, it was felt that it would be useful, in developing an overall picture of research ethics committees in Great Britain, to survey those in England and Wales. An immediate problem became apparent: whereas the Chief Scientist in the Scottish Home and Health Department had a list of research ethics committees in Scotland, no similar list for England and Wales was kept by the Department of Health and Social Security. The British Medical Association had undertaken its own survey[46] of the composition of research ethics committees in England and Wales in 1980, to which 73 out of 98 area medical officers had replied. The BMA's information, as well as being incomplete, would also have been out-of-date following the 1982 reorganization of the National Health Service, when area health authorities were abolished.

The research fellow therefore wrote, between December 1982 and February 1983, to the administrators of (a) the 192 English and 9 Welsh health districts, (b) the regional health authorities, (c) the postgraduate teaching hospitals, (d) the Royal Colleges, and (e) the Medical Research Council. The purpose of the survey was explained, and a prepaid envelope was provided, with a form requesting the names of any ethics committees within the domain of the administrator and the names of their chairmen. Reminder letters with a further form and pre-paid envelope were sent after a month. Eventually, all except 5 district administrators replied. A further 5 district administrators gave a nil return, in 2 cases because the ethics committees within their district were still being reorganized, and in 3 cases because there was no research ethics committee, its function being undertaken by a district medical committee or medical executive committee. One district administrator refused, on the advice of medical members of his district research ethics committee, to provide the name of the chairman of the committee.

The administrators identified a total of 254 research ethics committees. An explanatory letter was sent to the chairman of each committee. Two weeks later, in March 1983, a copy of the questionnaire was sent to each chairman with a prepaid envelope for its return; a further copy was sent to non-respondents after six weeks, and a reminder letter after a further six weeks. Completed questionnaires were returned for 174 (69 per cent) of the research ethics committees. Replies refusing to complete the questionnaire were received from 8 chairmen (3 per cent). The group of researchers served by the total number of research ethics committees, and by those that responded are compared in Table 8.1. It is apparent that the chairmen of research ethics committees who returned questionnaires are distributed amongst the categories of research ethics

committees in very similar proportions to those originally identified. The figure for chairmen who indicated that their committees
served only a hospital includes several whom the administrators
thought to be serving a district.

Table 8.1   Research ethics committees — replies to questionnaire

	Committees identified	Questionnaires returned
Research ethics committees serving:		
Part or whole district	158	101
Hospital	34	31
District containing teaching hospital	28	18
Single medical speciality within hospital or district	16	12
Hospital+research institute	11	10
Royal college	3	1
Research institute	2	1
Region	2	0
Totals	254	174

Results

Reference to the text of the questionnaire, in Appendix A, will indicate that each completed questionnaire contained a large
amount of information. The number of possible comparisons of
one variable in the combined results from all the returned questionnaires with any other variable is obviously enormous. In order to
try to extract as much useful information as possible about the
ways in which the committees work, four new variables were created to describe attributes of the committees and will be used
throughout the following pages. The first new variable is committee size: committees have been described as small, medium or
large if their total membership is in the range 3–5, 6–9, or 10 or
more members respectively. The second new variable is committee
workload: the committees have been divided according to whether
they received no research proposals at all in 1981 and 1982, 1 to 19
proposals in total (low workload) or 20 or more proposals (high

workload). The third new variable is very similar to the second, but considers the 'paediatric workload' caused by proposals for research on children only, dividing the committees into those that received no such proposals, those that received 1 to 3 proposals, and those that received 4 or more such proposals. The dividing points of 19 proposals in total and 3 proposals for research on children are the median values in each case for committee workload. The fourth variable to be created is the outcome of the review process. This is measured by the proportion of proposals for research on children, in 1981 and 1982, that a committee approved unchanged,

i.e.

$$\text{Outcome} = \frac{\text{Number of proposals approved unchanged}}{\text{Total child proposals} - \text{Withdrawn proposals}} \times 100 \text{ per cent.}$$

Outcome has been categorized as low when less than 60 per cent, medium when 61 to 99 per cent and high when 100 per cent. These four new variables have been compared with many of the other results of the survey in order to indicate how research ethics committees appear to function.

Authority of committee

One hundred and fifty-three chairmen (88 per cent of the 174 respondents) replied that it was compulsory for all proposals for research on human subjects within the relevant hospital, district, etc., to be submitted to the committee for approval. Of the 21 who said that it was not compulsory, only 7 provided written guidance to researchers on the categories of research that should be submitted. Those chairmen who said that it was compulsory were asked who had made the rule and gave the replies in Table 8.2.

[*Comment:* The replies in Table 8.2 suggest that some chairmen have no clear idea of the source of their authority: this would apply in particular to the chairmen who gave the replies in lines 6 to 9. When the research ethics committee (line 5) itself makes the rule for compulsory submission of all proposals, such a rule could only be effective if the committee had been asked to make its own rules by, for instance, the district health authority. The working group discussed at some length the accountability of research ethics committees: it concluded that they should be accountable in a fiduciary manner to the bodies that had established them, but that they should be responsible for protecting the interests both of research subjects and investigators. It should be noted that, of those chair-

Table 8.2   Source of authority of the committee

1.	Medical committee*	60	(39%)
2.	District health authority	22	(14%)
3.	District management team	9	(6%)
4.	Board of governors	8	(5%)
5.	The research ethics committee	13	(8%)
6.	Former area health authority or hospital management committee	9	(6%)
7.	Tradition/custom/consensus	6	(4%)
8.	'The consultants'	1	(1%)
9.	Not known	21	(14%)
10.	No reply	4	(3%)
	Total	153	(100%)

*'Medical committee' includes:
District medical committee
Medical advisory committee
Medical executive committee
Medical staff committee

men with a clear source of authority, only 30 derive that authority from a body that includes lay members (lines 2 and 4) while twice as many derive it from a medical committee.]

Chairmen were asked also whether they had become aware of any research projects being carried out in 1981 and 1982 within their 'jurisdiction', for which ethical approval had not been sought. Nineteen committees (12 per cent) had become aware of such research; in 9 cases one project had been discovered, in 6 cases two projects, and in 4 cases the number of projects discovered was not specified. Sixteen of the 19 committees had compulsory submission of projects, and 3 had not, a distribution very similar to the overall numbers of committees with or without compulsory submission.

Membership of the committee

The size of the research ethics committees varied considerably, although not quite so much as that of those in Scotland.[39] Committees in England and Wales ranged in size from 3 to 41 members, whereas those in Scotland ranged from 1 to 73 members! The mean size of committee was 8.4 members with a standard deviation of 5.7, and the commonest size was 5 members – the size of 31 committees (18 per cent). Forty-nine committees (28 per cent) had 10 or more members. The membership of the committees was, for the purposes of this study, divided into five categories: paediatricians or paediatric sub-specialists, general practitioners, others medically qualified, nurses, and 'others'. The average composition of each research ethics committee is shown in Table 8.3. While the overall mean figures may give some idea of the composition of the committees, the modal values may give a better impression of typical small (3–5 members), medium (6–9 members) or large (10 or more members) committees. The modal values are those which occurred most frequently in each group. The British Medical Association published its suggestions for the composition of research ethics committees in 1981;[46] its Council approved a revised

Table 8.3 Membership of the committees

	Survey results				BMA Models	
	Overall mean	Modal values			1981	1984
		small	medium	large		
Paediatricians	0.6	0	0	1	0	0
GPs	0.8	0	1	1	2	2
Other doctors	4.8	3	3	6	4	5
Nurses	0.6	0	1	1	1	1
'Others'	1.6	1	1	2	1	2
	8.4	4	6	11	8	10
Number of committees	174	63	62	49		

version[47] of these suggestions in 1984, but it has yet to be published.

Both the mean and modal values for committee composition disguise some other important figures. One hundred and eighteen (68 per cent) of the committees have no paediatrician at all, while exactly one-quarter (26) of all the paediatricians reported were members of the committee at one children's hospital. So just under one-third of all committees have a paediatrician member. Eighteen of the committees with no paediatrician had a high paediatric workload, i.e. reviewed 4 or more proposals for research on children in 1981 and 1982, and 28 committees without a paediatrician had a low paediatric workload, i.e. 1 to 3 proposals; information was available for 102 of the 118 committees with no paediatrician. Seventy-six (44 per cent) of the committees had no general practitioner member; 23 (13 per cent) had 2 or more general practitioners and would therefore meet the requirements of the British Medical Association's suggested composition for research ethics committees. The number of other doctors on the committees ranged from none to 38. Those committees with no other doctors served either children's hospitals or dental hospitals. The committee with 38 other doctors also had two paediatricians as members, so that its total composition was 40 hospital doctors and one lay person. Eighty-six (49 per cent) of the committees had no nursing members and only 8 (4.6 per cent) had two or more nurses.

[*Comment:* There has been ample illustration earlier in this report of the special problems of clinical research on children. These problems need to be presented to, and understood by, a research ethics committee. The obvious way in which to do this is by having a paediatrician as a member of the committee. In the absence of such membership, the fact that close to half such committees do consider proposals for research on children is a powerful argument in favour of committees co-opting paediatricians or other specialists who can inform their deliberations.]

Lay membership

The principle of having lay membership of research ethics committees seems to have been fairly generally accepted in that only 14 (8 per cent) of the committees have no 'other' members. Nine of these 14 committees have no nurse either, and were therefore composed entirely of doctors. The highest number of members of any committee who had qualifications neither in medicine nor in nursing was 7, but quite the most common number of such lay members was one: 93 committees, or 53 per cent of those replying, had a solitary lay member. In having a single lay member such committees are following the old recommendations of both the Royal College of Physicians[13] and the British Medical Association.[46] As was seen in Table 8.3, however, the revised BMA recommendation is for 2 lay members of research ethics committees, and the most recent Royal College of Physicians' *Guidelines on the practice of ethics committees in medical research*[48] suggest that membership 'should comprise at least . . . one, or perhaps better, two persons not trained in or practising any medical or paramedical discipline.' The study of research ethics committees in 'teaching districts' under-taken in 1981[40] showed that those committees on average had 2 lay members. This finding was confirmed in the present survey: while the average number of lay members for all committees was 1.6, the average for committees serving teaching hospitals and hospitals with research institutes was 2.3. Table 8.4 shows the occupations or professions of the 271 lay committee members for whom such information was given.

Table 8.4   Lay members

	Number	Percentage of total lay members
Member or chairman of Community Health Council	49	18
Health Service Administrator	35	13
Representative of Health Authority or Board of Governors	35	13
Lawyer	28	10.5
Clergyman	20	7.5
Non-clinical academic	15	5.5
Pharmacist	13	5
Businessman	10	4
Dentist/oral surgeon	9	3
Psychologist	9	3
Medical physicist/Laboratory Scientific Officer	8	3
Magistrate	7	2.5
Representative of local authority	6	2
Teacher	6	2
Other paramedical worker	5	2
Other 'lay' people (including architect, housewife, librarian, surveyor)	16	6

Although the principle of lay membership of research ethics committees may have been accepted, the purpose of such membership is by no means certain. The Proposed International Guidelines[15] suggest that laymen should be 'qualified to represent community, cultural and moral values'. Ryan, in discussing Institutional Review Boards in the US,[49] states that 'The layman is on the board to broaden the perspectives of the board on community attitudes and concerns and to call the professional's attention to incomprehensible consent forms.' Federal regulations in the US, in fact, specify that one member of each IRB must be independent, i.e. have no affiliation directly, or through a relative, with the institution. Such a requirement would probably not be met by 114 (42 per cent) of the lay members listed in Table 8.4. The Department of Health and Social Security guidelines in 1975[38] suggested that a suitable lay person would be a representative of the local Community Health Council, which presumably explains why such representatives constitute the largest group of lay members. Yet a paper discussing the Durham Area Ethical Committee[50] states that 'it was decided not to invite representation from the community health councils because it was felt that to involve council members in executive decision making would prejudice their otherwise unique roles as independent commentators upon the National Health Service.' Such a view is debatable: the 'executive decision-making' remains advisory in nature and lacks legal force. Moreover, representatives of community health councils are much more likely than most members of the public to have a good grasp both of medical vocabulary and the workings of the National Health Service, which could enhance their effectiveness in representing the community outside the institution to the other members of the committee.

One striking difference in lay membership between this survey and one carried out in the USA is in the number of lawyers. Gray *et al.* reported[51] that 'about three-fourths of the IRBs included a lawyer' when they surveyed 61 institutions in the USA. The present survey showed that only 16 per cent of research ethics committees have a lawyer as a lay member. One category of membership that was, surprisingly, completely absent was that of statistician: not a single committee reported a statistician amongst its membership. In this respect the finding is the same as in Gray's US survey: indeed the value of statistical advice is seldom mentioned in discussions of the role of institutional review boards.

In neither the United Kingdom nor in the United States of America has the question of lay membership been taken as seriously as in Denmark. In that country there are seven regional 'scientific-ethical' committees, each of which has six members and six substitutes, with an equal number of investigators and lay members in each group.[22] The lay members are appointed by the county councils. It was suggested to this working group that there is no intrinsic reason why research ethics committees in this country should have the preponderance of medically qualified members found in this survey and recommended by the British Medical Association and the Royal College of Physicians. In trying to decide what should be the proportion of lay members to others, one must ask what skills or experience each member of a committee may bring to it. In addition to the specialist advice that they may offer on issues concerning consent, lawyers are often experienced in understanding quickly the core of a variety of abstruse problems. Another sort of specialist advice may be available if a statistician can provide advice either as a consultant, or as a lay member of a committee: Altman[52] has recently discussed the ways in which statistically substandard research may be unethical. There are two more general functions that all lay members of research ethics committees need to carry out. One is to ensure that an investigator or group of investigators do not lose touch with the normally accepted standards of behaviour in the world outside the institution. The other is to place themselves, and by so doing make other members of the committee place themselves, in the position of a potential research subject: they can then ask whether they would wish the proposed research to be carried out on themselves or their families, and if so, what information they would wish to have. If lay members are to fulfil such functions, it is important that those who appoint them should choose people who are not likely to be intimidated by the medical members of the committee. The medical members, although not necessarily competent to judge the scientific value of a proposal, must be able to understand it and what it will entail for research subjects, and be able to interpret this to other members of the committee. The amount of knowledge now available about each medical specialty means that a member of one specialty may well understand little of another specialty, particularly at its research frontiers. Thus, it becomes necessary to have several medical members; experienced nurses may also be valuable members since they are more likely than either medical or lay members to be able to assess precisely what a project will entail in practice for the research subjects.

The foregoing does not allow one to draw any definite conclusions about the most desirable composition of a research ethics committee. The working group has recommended a possible constitution such that an ethics committee would have four hospital doctors, at least one general practitioner, at least one nurse and at least two lay members. In view of the potential for members to learn about research ethics, it is also suggested that in institutions where there are several doctors of registrar or senior registrar status involved in research, one such 'junior researcher' should be a member. The composition of any individual committee must depend, however, on the local availability of individuals who are not only competent to serve but are willing to work together with other committee members. Thus, one committee with a preponderance of lay members might work perfectly well, while another with a solitary lay member might be equally effective, because of the skills and effort that he was able to contribute. In general, however, the functions of the lay member require that there be at least two such members, who should be members in their own right and not representatives of a particular organization or viewpoint.

Other committee features

Chairmen of the committees were asked how many members of their committees had professional or expert experience of working with children, and how many members had particular experience in, or had made a special study of, ethical analysis or moral reasoning (see Appendix A for the examples given). Overall, 38 per cent of committees had no members with particular experience of working with children; 90 per cent of large committees, with 10 or more members, however, had such a member. Sixty per cent had no members with particular experience in ethical analysis: there was no significant difference between small and large committees in the numbers having such members.

The term of service of committee members was unspecified in 67 per cent of committees. In those committees in which a term was specified, it ranged from one year to ten, with a mean of 3.5 years. Fifty-six per cent of committees did not provide any briefing for their new members: large committees were more likely to do so than small committees, but the difference was not statistically significant.

Committee procedures

Various aspects of committee procedures that were primarily

administrative were examined in the questionnaire. Chairmen were asked whether they encouraged informal approaches by researchers prior to their submission of formal research proposals: 73 per cent do so. Fifty-two committees (30 per cent) have a standard application form for research proposals, and only 3 committees have a form specifically for research proposals on children. Large committees and those with a high workload, whether of total proposals or proposals for research on children, are all significantly more likely to have application forms. A curious, but statistically highly significant, finding was that committees using application forms are four times more likely to have a member of a health authority as a lay member than committees not using application forms. Thirty-four committees (20 per cent) neither encourage informal approaches nor have an application form for research proposals.

[*Comment:* Tannenbaum,[53] reporting a survey of research on children in the United States, found that 31 per cent of a sample of 471 investigators had had informal discussions with members of institutional review boards before submitting a formal proposal: over half of these discussions resulted in modifications to the proposal. It seems curious that, in the present survey, there were not 100 per cent of chairmen who encouraged informal approaches: not only can such approaches be extremely useful in giving an investigator a clear idea of the requirements of the committee, but they may also ensure that all necessary information is supplied to the committee, thus saving time for the committee and the investigator. A standard application form is another method of achieving much the same purpose. When a committee uses neither method, one can imagine that investigators must find it extremely difficult at times to know what sort of information the committee requires. Such a committee may in turn find its decisions more difficult to make because of missing or inappropriate information in submitted proposals. A specimen application form, based on various application forms supplied to this working group, is to be found in Appendix B.]

Twelve committees (7 per cent) do not normally circulate research proposals to each member of the committee. Whether or not all committee members have voting rights, it is a little difficult to see how such a practice can lead to worthwhile discussion by all committee members of research proposals. Most committees conduct their business either by meeting (52 per cent) or by post and by meeting (37 per cent). Ten committees (6 per cent) conduct their business by post only, while the remaining 8 (5 per cent) use other means, generally a mixture of the post and telephone. There was no significant difference in the ways committees conduct their business when considering proposals for research on children. The number of times that committees had met in the years 1981 and 1982 ranged from zero to 25 in each year, with a mean of 4 meetings per year. Chairmen were asked what percentage of members attended meetings on average, and the replies ranged from 35 to 100 per cent, with the latter being the most common value. As might be expected, large committees generally reported a slightly lower average attendance than small committees.

Sixty-seven chairmen answered a question asking how much time elapses, on average, between the first submission of a proposal for research on children, and the committee's final decision: the answers ranged from 2 to 13 weeks, with a mean of 5.6 weeks. Thirty-seven committees (55 per cent) took 4 weeks or less, while 20 committees (30 per cent) took 7 weeks or more to produce a decision. Large committees took on average 1.3 weeks less to produce a decision than small or medium committees: this probably reflects the fact that large committees hold more than twice as many meetings each year on average as small or medium committees (6.4 meetings per year compared to 3.1 meetings per year). Chairmen were also asked whether approval for proposals for research on children could be given either by the chairman alone or by a sub-committee. Eleven chairmen (7 per cent of those responding) could give such approval and 14 sub-committees (10 per cent).

[*Comment:* The regulations made by the Department of Health and Human Services in the USA allow ethical review by the chairman alone, or by one or more experienced reviewers designated by the chairman from the members of an Institutional Review Board. This process is known as 'expedited review' and is available for projects posing no more than minimal risk to the subjects (negligible risk in the BPA guidelines). The general categories of research for which expedited review is permissible are studies of substances obtained non-invasively – excreta, hair, nail-clippings, or expelled placentas – recordings by body-surface sensors, voice recordings, moderate exercise by healthy volunteers, and the use of surveys or psychological tests on normal volunteeers. Expedited review in no way removes from the researcher the obligation to submit projects of no more than minimal risk for ethical review.[54] But it does help to avoid the delays in ethical review that so often seem to cause investigators, and particularly those on relatively short-term appointments, to complain about the process. Thirty per cent of the chairmen replying in this survey said that ethical review, on average, took 7 weeks or longer. It is inevitable that researchers wanting to undertake the sort of projects listed above might find such a delay unreasonable. Expedited review, whether by the chairman or a sub-committee of the research ethics committee should become a far more commonly accepted practice in the United Kingdom.]

Chairmen were asked whether there had been any specific discussion in their committees, or in the group of researchers served, of the particular problems of research on children. Fifty (29 per cent) replied that there had been such discussion. Large committees and those with a high workload of proposals for research on children were more likely to have had such discussion. Chairmen were also asked for their opinions as to the usefulness of some of the guidelines mentioned already in this report: the Medical Research Council statement in 1963[7] (MRC), the Royal College of Physicians report in 1973[13] (RCP), the Department of Health and Social Security's Circular in 1975[38] (DHSS), the British Paediatric

Table 8.5 Opinions of guidelines

	Very helpful	Helpful	Unhelpful	Chairman unaware of existence	Committee aware of existence, but had no discussion
MRC	15.7	34.3	0.7	15.7	33.6
RCP	19.4	37.5	0.7	11.5	30.9
DHSS	10.7	37.1	1.4	18.6	32.2
BPA	14.7	16.2	0	29.4	39.7
WMA	16.7	36.1	2.1	9.0	36.1

(Figures in percentages for each guideline)

Association's 1980 guidelines[55] (BPA), and the 1975 revision of the Helsinki Declaration[6] (WMA). The replies are given in Table 8.5.

There appears to be little difference between knowledge of, and evaluation of usefulness of, the MRC, RCP, DHSS, and WMA guidelines. Those of the Royal College of Physicians and the

Helsinki Declaration are marginally better known and useful than the other two. But the British Paediatric Association guidelines, although published in the *British Medical Journal* as well as paediatric journals, are significantly ($p < 0.001$) less well known or discussed than the other four sets of guidelines. Fortunately, the ignorance of the BPA guidelines was greatest amongst the committees not reviewing research on children: 88 per cent of committees that received no proposals for research on children in 1981 and 1982 either had not discussed the BPA guidelines or had chairmen who were unaware of their existence; the figure for committees that had received proposals for research on children was 54 per cent. There was considerable overlap between the committees which had not discussed the particular problems of research on children and those that were unaware of, or had not discussed, the BPA guidelines. Seventy-five committees (55 per cent of the respondents) were in both categories.

The questionnaire produced one final and curious item about committee procedures: 5 committees either allocate funds for research, or make recommendations for such allocation to other committees. It is hard to see how such an activity can be considered proper for a research ethics committee, since it is so likely to produce conflicts of interest and purpose. At a meeting of the chairmen of teaching hospitals' research ethics committees held at the Royal College of Physicians in London in September 1982, there was virtually unanimous agreement that research ethics committees should have nothing to do with funding.

Proposals for research on children

Chairmen were asked how many proposals in total their committees had received in the two-year period 1981–2, and the outcome of the review of proposals for research on children. Since it was thought that some chairmen would not have ready access to the necessary figures, they were invited to estimate the figures rather than not to answer the questions. Only 20 (13 per cent) of the figures for proposals for research on children were estimates; when compared with the overall figures for means and standard deviations, there were no significant differences, and so the combined figures have been used in this analysis.

The total number of proposals for research on adults and children reviewed by each committee in the two-year period ranged from 0 (14 committees) to 346, with a mean of 41 projects. The number of proposals for research on children ranged from 0 (65 committees – 42 per cent) to 125, with a mean of 4.3 proposals reviewed by each committee over the two years. This figure allows one to produce an approximate estimate of the number of children involved in clinical research in England and Wales each year.

If one assumes that those committees for which a questionnaire was not completed reviewed on average as many proposals for research on children as the committees that did respond, then the total number of such proposals in the two-year period would have been 4.3×254, where 254 is the number of research ethics committees identified in this survey in England and Wales. This would give a total of 1092 projects, but previous reports suggest that about 10 per cent of proposals either do not receive ethics committee approval, are withdrawn, or are never started. It would therefore be a reasonable approximation to suggest that 1000 projects on children might have been started in the two-year period 1981–2. The journal *Archives of Disease in Childhood* has been reviewed for 1983 in order to assess how many child subjects are entered into research projects. Only reports of research carried out in the United Kingdom were considered, and any reports of population screening were excluded. Eighty-eight research projects were reported, the number of subjects ranging from 1 to 655; the mean number of subjects was 90.1 with 95 per cent confidence limits of 64.0 and 116.2. If the average number of subjects of research projects reported in this journal is taken to be the average for all projects on children in England and Wales, then approximately 90 000 children will be involved in clinical research projects in a two year period. The child population of England and Wales is approximately 12 000 000, so 0.75 per cent of all children are likely to be involved in clinical research in a two-year period. Put another way, 6 per cent of children, or one child in every seventeen, are likely to be the subjects of clinical research during their childhood.

A total of 659 proposals for research on children were reported to have been received by 155 committees and information about the outcome of 645 proposals was also available: it is given in Table 8.6. One hundred and forty proposals (21 per cent) were rejected by the committees or modified at their request, while 75 per cent were approved unchanged. This may be compared with the results of several studies as shown in Table 8.7: it should be noted that the other studies were all of proposals for research on both adults and children.

Table 8.6   Outcome of proposals for research on children

Total proposals	659	
Rejected outright	8	1%
Modified substantially	24	4%
Modified slightly	108	16%
Approved unchanged	493	75%
Withdrawn by applicant	12	2%
Outcome unknown	14	2%

Table 8.7   Approval rates reported for various ethical review committees

Place	Year	Total proposals	Approved unchanged
Newcastle[44]	1972–6	249	86%
Harrow[43]	1970–8	580	70%
Southampton[41]	1971	30	90%
	1975	67	75%
	1979	44	61%
Scotland[39]	1979	370	84%
USA[51]	1974–5	2389	44%
England and Wales (Present study)	1981–2	659	75%

The outcome of proposals for research on children is related in Table 8.8 to the size of the committees reviewing the proposals, and to the total number of proposals reviewed. It is apparent that large committees generally had many more proposals submitted to them than small or medium committees. This point is exemplified by the histogram in Fig. 8.1; but it should be noted both that some large committees received no proposals at all for research on children and that some small committees had a high paediatric workload. Table 8.8 shows an association between the size of a committee and the number of proposals for research on children that were approved unchanged: large committees approved a significantly higher proportion of proposals unchanged.

An association was sought between the presence on a committee of a paediatrician, a 'child expert', or a 'moralist' and the outcome

Table 8.8   Size of committee and outcome of proposals (1981–1982)

Committee size	Small	Medium	Large
Number of members	3–5	6–9	10 or more
Number of committees	63 (36%)	62 (36%)	49 (28%)
Total proposals	732	1646	3586
Total proposals per committee	11.6	26.6	73.2
Proposals for research on children	84	130	445
Child research proposals per committee	1.3	2.1	9.1
Child research proposals as proportion of total research proposals	11.5%	7.9%	12.4%
Outcome of child research proposals:			
(a) Rejected	0	2	6
(b) Substantially modified	1	5	18
(c) Slightly modified	31	32	45
(d) Rejected or modified	32 (38%)	39 (30%)	69 (16%)
(e) Approved unchanged	51 (61%)	71 (55%)	371 (83%)
(f) Withdrawn	0	7	5
(g) Outcome unknown	1	13	0

of proposals for research on children. One might have expected that the presence of a member in any of these categories would make it more likely that a proposal for research on children would be thoroughly scrutinized, and thus more often be rejected or, in particular, modified. Table 8.9 illustrates that the presence of such members appears to have the opposite effect. The presence of either a paediatrician, a 'child expert' or a 'moralist' on a research ethics committee made it significantly more likely that proposals for research on children would be approved unchanged. It is important to note, however, that committees with members in these categories examine, on average, between twice and five times as many proposals as committees without such membership. These results may therefore just reflect a rather similar result to that shown in Table 8.8 – that committees with a higher workload tend to approve more proposals unchanged.

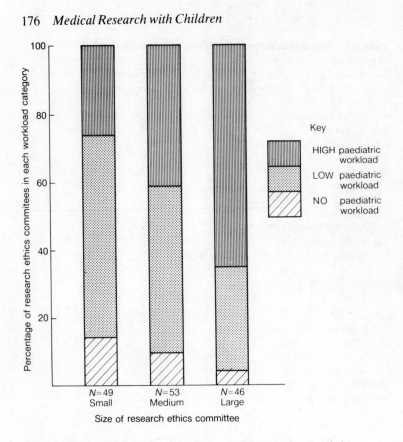

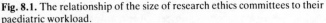

Fig. 8.1. The relationship of the size of research ethics committees to their paediatric workload.

Committee performance

Tables 8.8 and 8.9, as well as producing slightly unexpected results, represent rather a crude assessment of the outcome of proposals for research on children, since the results for all committees have been lumped together. As mentioned previously (p.161), a measure of the outcome of each individual committee's review process has therefore been developed. The outcome for an individual committee is the number of proposals approved unchanged as a percentage of the total number of proposals for research on children that were either approved, modified or rejected. Committees have then been categorized as having a low outcome when less than 60 per cent of proposals were approved unchanged, a medium outcome for 61 to 99 per cent, and a high outcome when all proposals

Table 8.9 Association between various members of committee and outcome of proposals for research on children

	Number of proposals* (percentage)	
	Rejected/ modified	Approved unchanged
Committee having:		
(1) Paediatrician member	73 (17%)	357 (83%)
No paediatrician member	67 (33%)	136 (67%)
(2) 'Child expert'† member	112 (20%)	446 (80%)
No 'child expert' member	28 (37%)	47 (63%)
(3) 'Moralist'§ member	64 (18%)	288 (82%)
No 'moralist' member	76 (27%)	205 (73%)

Notes: *Number of proposals excludes those withdrawn and those with unknown outcome.
†'Child expert': someone with professional or expert experience of working with children: see Appendix A for examples.
§'Moralist': someone with particular experience in, or who has made a special study of, ethical analysis or moral reasoning: see Appendix A for examples.

Table 8.10 Outcome v. committee size

	Number of committees		
Outcome	Small (3–5 members)	Medium (6–9 members)	Large (10 or more members)
Low (0–60%)	9	11	5
Medium (61–99%)	4	4	14
High (100%)	14	11	15
No applications	25	26	14

were approved unchanged; a fourth category includes committees that received no proposals for research on children.

Table 8.10 shows the relationship of outcome for individual committees to the size of the committees. A trend can still be discerned towards a higher level of approval unchanged of proposals submitted to large committees, but it is no longer significant. On the other hand, Table 8.11 shows a highly significant distinction between the outcomes for committees with high and low paediatric workloads: 66 per cent of committees with a low paediatric workload approved all proposals for research on children, but only 23 per cent of those with a high paediatric workload did so.

Table 8.11   Outcome v. paediatric workload

Outcome	Committees in each category of paediatric workload		
	None	Low (1–3)	High (4 or more)
Low (0–60%)		12	13
Medium (61–99%)		4	18
High (100%)		31	9
No applications	65		

[*Comment:* When individual committee performance is examined, it becomes apparent that the association between large committee size and high approval rate is much less secure. Indeed, since the tendency has been shown for large committees to have a high workload and small committees a low workload, the results of Table 8.11 are contrary to expectations. One must look for another explanation for these results: perhaps the most realistic is to suggest that committees that only occasionally review proposals for research on children may have less experience and expertise in detecting shortcomings in them and in suggesting improvements.]

The same categories of membership of a research ethics committee as were considered earlier – 'child expert', 'moralist', or paediatrician – have been related to outcome in Table 8.12, as have the other categories of membership for which information was available. The figures show no significant difference between the outcomes for committees with or without a paediatrician, a general practitioner, a 'child expert' or a 'moralist'. There is a trend towards a lower outcome when there is a lay member of a committee but the number of committees without a lay member is too small for this trend to be significant. The one significant result is that committees with nurse members are less likely to approve all proposals for research on children than committees without a nurse member.

[*Comment:* These results provide no evidence of any association between most categories of committee membership and the outcome of consideration of proposals for research on children. They do, however, provide the basis of a strong argument for the value

Table 8.12   Outcome v. membership of committees

Committees having:	Low (0–60%)	Medium (61–99%)	High (100%)	No proposals
1. No paediatrician	13	11	22	56
Paediatrician member	12	11	18	9
2. No general practitioner	10	6	18	29
GP member	15	16	22	36
3. No nurse	10	4	26	34
Nurse member	15	18	14	31
4. No 'child expert'	4	3	9	36
'Child expert' member	21	19	31	27
5. No 'moralist'	16	10	22	38
'Moralist' member	9	12	18	26
6. No lay member	0	1	6	5
Lay member	25	21	34	60

of having a nurse as a member of a research ethics committee. The fact that only 30 per cent of committees with a nurse member approve all proposals unchanged, compared to 65 per cent of committees without a nurse member, suggests that a nurse can provide a valuable degree of scrutiny of proposals.]

One further indication of committee performance is provided by the association between outcome and discussion of research on children. The questionnaire asked committee chairmen whether there had been 'any specific discussion in the committee, or in the group of researchers it serves, of the particular problems of research on children?' Table 8.13 shows that when such discussion had taken place a committee was significantly less likely to approve all proposals unchanged.

[*Comment:* It would be nice to suggest that Table 8.13 is demonstrating a cause-and-effect relationship – that discussion of the problems of research on children leads to greater awareness of those problems, more thorough scrutiny of proposals and thus a higher modification and rejection rate – but, even with a high degree of statistical significance, one could not claim to have proved such a relationship. Moreover, there are examples of committees for whom the benefit of having prior discussion of the problems of re-

Table 8.13   Outcome v. discussion of research on children

Outcome	Discussion	
	Yes	No
Low (0–60%)	17	8
Medium (61–99%)	12	10
High (100%)	11	29
No proposals	7	57

search on children has evidently been outweighed by other constraints imposed by the structure of the committee. One committee, for instance, had 39 members, including paediatricians, other 'child experts' and a 'moralist'. In 1981 and 1982 they considered a total of 71 proposals; of these 27 were for research on children, and all 27 were approved unchanged. The chairman reported an average attendance of 75 per cent at the committee's monthly meetings: common sense – and communication theory in social psychology – would surely indicate that meetings of a committee with an average attendance of 30 are likely to be less efficient or effective than the meetings of a smaller committee. There may also be an additional problem when a committee has large numbers of consultants as members (this committee included 33 hospital doctors); there may be an increased reluctance to comment on or criticize each other's work in such a public forum. A similar problem may explain why the presence of a paediatrician as a committee member appears to have little effect on the outcome of a committee's review of proposals for research on children. Most committees with paediatric membership have a single paediatrician, and probably serve 'jurisdictions' within which there are at most two other paediatricians. Although a paediatrician may not always be named as principal investigator, one of them is likely to be involved in each project in one way or another – whether as investigator, supervisor, or source of subjects. If that one is a member of the research ethics committee the other members may not wish to criticize his project; if he is not, then the paediatrician who is on the committee may likewise not wish to criticize his colleague's proposal.]

These reflections may be used to illustrate a general comment on the work of research ethics committees. There has been general approval both in the United Kingdom and the United States of America for establishing ethical review committees close to where the research to be reviewed will take place, and preferably within the same institution. In particular, it has been suggested that the personal knowledge that the members of the committees will have of the investigators will assist the committee members in reviewing the research proposals. Proximity of the committee members and investigators can also promote informal discussion of projects, and assist committee members in following up their decisions and recommendations should they wish to do so. It is evident, however, that such proximity may have drawbacks. Unless committee members are extremely careful, ties of friendship and professional collaboration may cause them to be less than objective, and possibly to fail in their role of protecting research subjects. Proximity and the opportunity for informal discussion may also explain, in part, the higher rate of approval of proposals by larger committees. It could be postulated that the larger a committee the greater its educational effect in the 'jurisdiction' that it serves, since more members will presumably mean a greater number of opportunities for discussion of the requirements of the committee. This could explain the decreasing rate of rejection and modification as committees become larger. There might also be an 'educational' effect working in the opposite direction. In institutions with a high level of research activity, a research ethics committee member will be more likely to have observed research projects that have provided highly beneficial results. It is possible that such experience might make the committee member more directly in favour of research as an enterprise than if he had not had such experience; and thus more likely to approve proposals put to the committee.

The questionnaire went on to ask committee chairmen the reasons for their decisions to reject or modify proposals for research on children. Of the eight rejected proposals, one was rejected for poor research design, one for inadequate arrangements for obtaining consent, and one for poor research design and ethical unacceptability. The remaining five were rejected because of ethical unacceptability. Reasons were also supplied for the committees' decisions to request modification for 125 of the total of 132 modified proposals. These are given in Table 8.14. The most common reasons mentioned under 'other problems' were lack of information or consultation. In some cases the researchers had given inadequate information to the research ethics committee, and in

Table 8.14   Reasons for request for slight or substantial modification of proposals for research on children

Total modified proposals	132
Reasons for modification:	
1. Poor research design	19 (14%)
2. Acceptable research design but lack of scientific value	7 (5%)
3. Ethical unacceptability	31 (23%)
4. Inadequate arrangements for obtaining consent	46 (35%)
5. Other problems	22 (17%)
6. Not specified	7 (5%)

others proposed to give inadequate information to the parents of subjects. Inadequate consultation with other interested disciplines was given as the reason for modification of two proposals, and failure to inform the subjects' general practitioners was given as the reason in several other cases. Only one proposal was mentioned in which the committee had asked the researcher to give the parents more time to make up their minds about giving or withholding consent. One committee, in an area with a large and generally non-English-speaking immigrant community, had asked for the modification of proposals in which there was a lack of awareness of their racial impact and a lack of provision for adequate communication with non-English speakers.

There are unfortunately almost no figures available with which to compare the information given here about the outcome of proposals for research on children. Tannenbaum and Cooke[53] interviewed researchers undertaking a total of 471 research projects on children in 1974 and 1975 in a survey undertaken for the National Commission for the Protection of Human Subjects of Biomedical and Behavioral Research in the United States of America. They recorded that ethical review committees had required modifications 'in regard to how consent would be obtained from subjects' in 25 per cent of the total number of projects. In the present survey, there were inadequate arrangements for obtaining consent in 46 proposals, and more time was requested for the consent procedure in another proposal. So modifications in the manner of gaining consent were requested in 47 proposals, or 7 per cent of the total. The most likely reason for such a discrepancy between English and American figures lies in the regulations by which institutional review boards in the USA have been established. The regulations specify the criteria for IRB approval of research, which include the requirement for informed consent not only to be sought from each research subject or his proxy, but also to be adequately documented. Thus, an IRB has a statutory duty to examine the process of gaining consent, and any consent forms that may be used.

Consent to research on children

The policies of research ethics committees on the obtaining of consent for research on children were examined further in the questionnaire. The responses to several questions are tabulated in Table 8.15. The most striking finding is the first one: 20 committees (18 per cent of the respondents) do not always insist on investigators obtaining consent from parents or guardians before their children may be entered into a research project.

[*Comment:* Although the legal concept of consent, either in routine medical practice or in research, is of relatively recent origin,[56] it is now widely accepted that the patient's consent, or that of someone with the legal right to speak for him, is required before a doctor may carry out a procedure on the patient. In the United Kingdom such consent need not always be explicit, but may be implied, as when a doctor touches a patient in order to examine him during a consultation that the patient has initiated by presenting himself to the doctor. When there is neither implicit nor explicit consent, the procedure is likely to be illegal, being an assault or trespass, except in well-defined circumstances such as emergencies. If the procedure is a research procedure, however, the doctor may not assume that consent is implied: research has never become so routine an activity. Thus, there must be an explicit consent for any research procedure, if it is to be legally performed. There may be a few exceptions to this general rule, as for instance in research that involves only observation of a child. The rule will apply, however, to research involving any sort of intervention, and most observations, if of individual children, will also require explicit consent. It seems likely that some of the 18 per cent of committees that do not always insist on parental consent provide ethical review for units and institutions such as the special care baby unit, mentioned earlier in the report, at which it has not been the policy to obtain informed consent from parents for research on their infants. Such a policy seems to result from too ready an acceptance of the apparent difficulties in obtaining consent from the parents of newborn children rather than from any argument that consent is not legally and ethically necessary. The problem of obtaining consent for research on newborn infants is discussed further in the next chapter.]

Fifteen per cent of committees do not always insist on parents or guardians being given a full explanation of research on their children, for which consent is being sought (Table 8.15, line 2).

[*Comment:* While it is well known that there can be considerable difficulties in providing an explanation of any sort in language which most parents could understand, the law nevertheless requires the attempt to be made, since consent which is not fully informed may be held to be invalid. Since two-thirds of the committees that do not always require a full explanation are committees which also do not always insist on consent being obtained from parents , the answers to these two questions suggest that approximately one committee in every ten is not aware of the legal need for fully informed consent to research procedures.]

The remaining questions listed in Table 8.15 refer to aspects of the process of gaining consent which have no legal implications in the United Kingdom, although some of them are covered by federal regulations in the United States of America. In neither country is there any requirement legally for a length of time to elapse between the giving of an explanation of a research project and the request for consent from the parents or guardians of a child to be entered into the project. Since more than two-thirds of research ethics committees never insist on such a pause, it is evident that it is not often thought necessary. Patients, however, or the parents of child patients, often feel under pressure to co-operate. Time for reflection away from the research setting would not only relieve such pressure, but would enable parents to assess just how much of an explanation they had understood and to work out what additional information they wanted before making a decision. It

Table 8.15   Policies for consent

	Numbers of respondents				Total
	Always	Usually	Sometimes	Never	
1. Does your committee insist that researchers gain consent from parents or guardians of a child before that child may be entered into a research project?	94	19	1	0	114
2. If consent is sought from parents or guardians, does your committee require them to be given a full explanation of the proposed research?	94	17	0	0	111
3. Does the committee insist that consent to research on children be obtained from the parents or guardians in writing?	47	25	26	8	106
4. Does the committee require the obtaining of consent to research on children to be witnessed by a 'third party'?	15	12	14	60	101
5. Does the committee insist that parents or guardians of child research subjects be given a copy in writing of:					
(a) the explanation of the research?	11	8	28	53	100
(b) the consent form?	14	7	19	58	98
6. Does the committee specify that a length of time should elapse between an explanation being given to parents or guardians, and the request for their consent?	7	12	13	70	102

seems reasonable to suggest that whenever research involving greater than a minor increase over minimal risk (American definition: see Chapter 5) is proposed on a child subject, there should be a pause of at least one day between an explanation being given to the child's parents or guardians and the request for consent. A research ethics committee could obviously allow exceptions to this rule if it appeared that research carrying the prospect of real benefit would be made impossible by such a rule.

The third line of Table 8.15 shows that two-thirds of the respondent committees always, or usually, require written consent to research on children, while just 8 committees never require written consent. Seven of the latter committees were also amongst the 60 committees who also never require the obtaining of consent to be witnessed (line 4). Although no relationship was found between the paediatric workload of a committee and its insistence on the gaining of parental consent, committees with a high paediatric workload were significantly less likely to insist on written consent than other committees: 28 per cent did so, compared with 56 per cent of other committees. However, the group of committees with a high paediatric workload was also significantly more likely to insist on consent being witnessed, either always or usually (40 per cent compared with 12 per cent).

[*Comment:* It is not certain that written consent has any general advantage over oral consent, since written consent in the absence of evidence that a full and truthful explanation has been given beforehand will be of as little value as unrecorded consent. Just as surgeons, however, feel legally better protected by the existence of written consent to the surgical procedures they carry out, so also researchers may gain similar benefit by obtaining written consent. In the United States, written consent is in general required for all research procedures other than those covered by the rules for expedited review – i.e. those of no more than minimal risk. If oral consent is obtained for research in the latter category, it must be witnessed by a third party who must record the obtaining of oral consent in writing. Obviously, one hopes that disputes about research will be rare, and never have to end in court. If they do so, a researcher is likely to be best protected by having obtained written consent and by having evidence of a full explanation having been given. The use of, for instance, a nurse – preferably of similar standing to the investigator: e.g. a ward sister – as a third party to witness both the explanation and the obtaining of consent is probably the simplest way of providing such evidence. Since a nurse is likely to have an understanding of a research project that lies between that of the investigator and that of the parent, the nurse can do much to ensure that the explanation is understood by the parent.

The questions in lines 3 to 6 of Table 8.15 relate to parts of the process of obtaining consent that are commonly carried out in the United States, in some cases, such as questions 5(a) and (b), because of federal regulations. Only a minority of research ethics committees in England and Wales insist on any of these parts of the process, other than the obtaining of written consent. Those committees that insist on one part of the process do not in general insist on the other parts. It is possible, however, to argue that all the parts of the process can be of considerable value to the parents of research subjects, even if researchers are worried by the possible addition to the time taken to obtain consent. It seems important therefore that research ethics committees should be aware of the possibilities – of requiring a pause between explanation and asking for consent, of requiring written consent, of requiring witnessed consent and of providing copies in writing of the explanation and consent form – so that they may insist on investigators using any or all of these parts of the process of obtaining consent when it is evident that parents or guardians would thus benefit.]

Questions were asked to discover who may give an explanation of a research project to the parents or guardians of a child research subject, and who is allowed to obtain consent from them. The answers are shown in Table 8.16 in terms of the percentage of committee chairmen who indicated that persons in each category could give an explanation or obtain consent.

Table 8.16 Persons involved in consent process

	Give explanation	Gain consent
The researcher	99%	98%
Another doctor	24%	40%
Ward sister	9%	11%
Any nurse	4%	2%
Others	6%	8%

[*Comment:* The results are fairly unremarkable, though some might be surprised at the number of committees that allow a ward sister or nurse both to explain and to obtain consent. If, however, the research is taking place in a unit in which the researcher and other staff work as a well-informed team, then it is quite possible that a nurse could give a better understood explanation than the researcher, and, naturally, continue on to obtain consent.]

Children's participation in consent

The final questions relating to the obtaining of consent that were asked concerned the involvement of child research subjects themselves in the process. Eighteen chairmen replied to the question 'From what age upwards, of a child research subject, does the committee require researchers to obtain the child's assent to a research procedure?' The replies ranged from 10 years to 17, with 16 the most common reply, and a mean of 14.3 years. Seven of the replies, however, were from chairmen of committees that had considered no proposals for research on children in 1981 and 1982. Those seven replies had a mean of 15.0 years as the age above which a child's assent is required, while the other eleven replies, from committees that had considered an average of 17 proposals each for research on children in the same period, gave a mean of 13.9 years, with 12 years the commonest age.

[*Comment:* Evidence was presented in the previous chapter that, while they were not fully competent, children in the age range 7 to 11 years were capable of making rational decisions about medical matters. Yet only one committee – that which gave 10 years as the age of assent – requires researchers to obtain assent from children in that age range.]

Rather more chairmen (41) replied to a question asking at what age the committees considered a child's consent to research to be sufficient by itself. The replies ranged from 14 to 18 years, the most frequent being 16 years, with a mean of 16.6 years.

[*Comment:* No distinction was made in the question between consent to therapeutic or to non-therapeutic research. Such a distinction may be important in that there seems to be good reason to suggest that consent to therapeutic research is legally valid from the age of 16 upwards, while consent to non-therapeutic research may not be legally valid until a person is 18 years old. If, on the other hand, one is considering the age at which a child is likely to be competent to give consent, then the answer from the previous chapter appears to be when he has reached a developmental age of 14 years.]

Monitoring

Since research ethics committees first developed, the main argument about their role has been whether it should be purely advisory or whether there should be a continuing involvement. The former view holds that the committees were set up on the advice of the Department of Health and Social Security and the Royal College of Physicians to provide a forum for peer review; the committees, having no statutory basis, are formal bodies that provide advice to researchers, from their colleagues, about the ethics of proposed research projects. The alternative view accepts the above as part of the role of a research ethics committee, but stresses also the purpose of the committee in providing protection for the subjects of the proposed research. Such protection could not be provided by a purely advisory role: it is necessary for the committee to monitor the progress of research projects. Heath has written[57] about four aspects of monitoring that institutional review boards in the United States might undertake, in part, at least, to satisfy federal regulations: (a) review of the way in which consent is actually being obtained; (b) review for adherence to the approved research protocol; (c) 'continuing review' to examine whether the results of the project itself or of other published new work significantly alter the need to continue the project; and (d) identification of research activities not approved by the IRB. Obviously, one of the main arguments against such activities in Great Britain is finding the time and personnel to do it: that it can be contemplated in the United States is probably a reflection of the fact that there is money available for a person like Heath to be employed as 'administrative analyst' to a committee on human research.

A few questions were asked in the survey about research ethics committees' monitoring, or follow-up. Forty-eight per cent of committees sometimes ask for a progress report on approved projects; unfortunately, the question was not designed to find out how frequently they do so. Similarly, 43 per cent sometimes ask for a final report on completion of an approved research project. The practice reported by the Northwick Park research ethics committee[43] was to send out a 'project review form' once each year asking about the numbers of subjects studied, any alterations in the protocol, any problems, particularly ethical, that had arisen and any planned future developments. The Southampton committee[41] sends out a similar questionnaire once every two years 'but not all are returned'. The use of annual review seems likely to provide research ethics committees with useful follow-up information while not necessarily making them appear too authoritarian.

Chairmen were asked whether their committees had ever received any complaints about research on children that they had approved. Only two such complaints had ever been received, in both cases from doctors. In one case the complaint had been based on a misunderstanding, while in the other, it was based on the lack of scientific value of a project coupled to the emotional distress caused to the children involved. One chairman reported having received complaints from several doctors about a project for research on children before his committee had considered it. He did not tell the committee of these complaints, and it rejected the project outright. Although these complaints form a tiny sample, it is interesting that all originated from doctors. It may well be that the most effective form of monitoring is for other doctors, particularly clinicians with clinical responsibility for research subjects, to be aware of what is happening to research subjects and to be willing to comment. On the other hand, it is unlikely that more than a very small proportion of the general public are even aware of the existence of research ethics committees. Perhaps such committees should attempt to publicize their own existence and purpose, so that, at the least, research subjects, or the parents of child research subjects, should be told about the committee and the possibility of submitting comments or complaints to it.

References

1. Levine, R.J. The value and limitations of ethical review committees for clinical research. In *Medical ethics and medical education* (eds. Z. Bankowski and J.C. Bernardelli) pp.43–63. CIOMS, Geneva (1981).
2. Percival, T. Medical ethics (1803). Reprinted in *Percival's medical ethics* (ed. C.D. Leake) pp.61–206 Krieger, Huntington, NY (1975).
3. German Reich. Circular of the Ministry of the Interior on directives concerning new medical treatments and scientific experiments on man (1931). Translated in *Int. Dig. Hlth Legisl. (Geneva)* **31**, 408–11 (1980).

4. Howard-Jones, N. Human experimentation in historical and ethical perspectives. In *Human experimentation and medical ethics* (eds. Z. Bankowski and N. Howard-Jones) pp.453–95. CIOMS, Geneva (1982).
5. The Nuremberg Code. Reprinted in *Dictionary of medical ethics* (2nd edn) (eds. A.S. Duncan, G.R. Dunstan, and R.B. Welbourn) pp.130–32. Darton, Longman, & Todd, London (1981).
6. World Medical Association. *Declaration of Helsinki:* Recommendations guiding physicians in biomedical research involving human subjects. (Adopted, Helsinki, 1964; amended, Tokyo, 1975 and Venice, 1983).
7. Medical Research Council. Responsibility in investigations on human subjects. In *Report of the Medical Research Council for the year 1962–63*, pp.21–5. HMSO, London (1964).
8. Curran, W.J. Governmental regulation of the use of human subjects in medical research: the approach of two federal agencies. In *Experimentation with human subjects* (ed. P.A. Freund) pp.402–54. George Allen & Unwin, London (1972).
9. The National Research Act (Public Law 93-348). Reprinted in *Protection of human research subjects* (ed. D.M. Maloney) pp.23–30. Plenum, New York (1984).
10. President's Commission for the Study of Ethical Problems in Medicine and Biomedical and Behavioral Research. *Implementing human research regulations.* US Government Printing Office, Washington DC (1983).
11. Welt, L. G. Reflections on the problems of human experimentation. *Connecticut Medicine* **25,** 75–9 (1961).
12. Barber, B., Lally, J., Makarushka, J.L., and Sullivan, D. *Research on human subjects: problems of social control in medical experimentation,* p.148. Transaction Books, New Brunswick, NJ (1979).
13. Royal College of Physicians. *Supervision of the ethics of clinical research investigations in institutions.* Royal College of Physicians, London (1973).
14. Pappworth, M.H. *Human guinea pigs,* p.252. Routledge & Kegan Paul, London (1967).
15. Council for International Organizations of Medical Sciences. *Proposed international guidelines for biomedical research involving human subjects.* CIOMS, Geneva (1982).
16. Department of Health and Human Services. Final regulations amending basic HHS policy for the protection of human research subjects (45CFR46) *Federal Register* **46**(16), 8366–91 (1981).
17. Pavlovsky, S. Clinical research and the protection of the subject in Argentina. In *Medical ethics and medical education* (eds. Z. Bankowski and J.C. Bernardelli) pp.118–23. CIOMS, Geneva (1981).
18. National Health and Medical Research Council. *Ethics in medical research.* Australian Government Publishing Service, Canberra (1983).

19. Freedman, B. Une expérience en éthique de l'expérimentation: les directives du Conseil de recherches médicales. In *Cahiers de bioéthique 4: Médecine et expérimentation* (eds. M.A.M. de Wachter, D.J. Roy, H. Doucet, and E. Baril) pp.139–60. Les Presses de L'Université Laval, Quebec (1982).

20. Canadian Medical Research Council. *Ethical considerations in research involving human subjects.* MRC, Ottawa (1978).

21. Brunser, O. An experience of protection of the research subject and clinical research in Chile. In *Medical ethics and medical education* (eds. Z. Bankowski and J.C. Bernardelli) pp.124–8. CIOMS, Geneva (1981).

22. Riis, P. Experiences with committees and councils for research ethics in Scandinavia. In *Research ethics* (eds. K. Berg and K.E. Tranoy) pp.123–9. Alan Liss, New York (1983).

23. Rouzioux, J-M. Les essais de nouveaux médicaments. In *Cahiers de bioéthique 4: Médecine et expérimentation* (eds. M.A.M. de Wachter, D.J. Roy, H. Doucet, and E. Baril) pp.161–70. Les Presses de L'Université Laval, Quebec (1982).

24. Indian Council of Medical Research. Policy statement on ethical considerations involved in research on human subjects. *Int. Dig. Hlth Legisl.* **31,** 980–6 (1980).

25. Gopalan, C. Ethical aspects in community-based research with particular emphasis on nutrition research. In *Human experimentation and medical ethics* (eds. Z. Bankowski and N. Howard-Jones) pp.124–43. CIOMS, Geneva (1982).

26. Soh, C-T. National drug regulations and ethical review procedures in Korea. In *Human experimentation and medical ethics* (eds. Z. Bankowski and N. Howard-Jones) pp.239–41. CIOMS, Geneva (1982).

27. Sinnathuray, T.A. Ethical review procedures in Malaysia. In *Human experimentation and medical ethics* (eds. Z. Bankowski and N. Howard-Jones) pp.235–8. CIOMS, Geneva (1982).

28. Ethical issues and professional responsibility: Mexico. *Int. Dig. Hlth Legisl.* **35,** 355–8 (1984).

29. Hodge, J.V. Ethical review procedures in New Zealand. In *Human experimentation and medical ethics* (eds. Z. Bankowski and N. Howard-Jones) pp.231–234. CIOMS, Geneva (1982).

30. Ajayi O.O. Taboos and clinical research in West Africa. *J. med. Ethics* **6,** 61–3 (1980).

31. Cortes-Maramba, N.P. Requirements for informed consent of subjects in the Philippines. In *Human experimentation and medical ethics* (eds. Z. Bankowski and N. Howard-Jones) pp.80–2. CIOMS, Geneva (1982).

32. Giertz, G. Ethical aspects of paediatric research. *Acta paediat. scand.* **72,** 641–50 (1983).

33. Zetterstrom, R. Ethical aspects of clinical trials design in Sweden. In *Human experimentation and medical ethics* (eds. Z. Bankowski and N. Howard-Jones) pp.242–5. CIOMS, Geneva (1982).

34. Greenwald, R.A., Ryan, M.K., and Mulvihill, J.E. (eds.) *Human subjects research: a handbook for institutional review boards.* Plenum, New York (1982).
35. Maloney, D.M. *Protection of human research subjects: a practical guide to Federal laws and regulations.* Plenum, New York (1984).
36. Levine, R.J. *Ethics and regulation of clinical research.* Urban & Schwarzenberg, Baltimore (1981).
37. Fluss, S.S. The proposed guidelines as reflected in legislation and codes of ethics. In *Human experimentation and medical ethics* (eds. Z. Bankowski and N. Howard-Jones) pp.323–66. CIOMS, Geneva (1982).
38. Department of Health and Social Security. *Supervision of the ethics of clinical research investigations and fetal research.* HSC (IS) 153, DHSS, London (1975).
39. Thompson, I.E., French, K., Melia, K.M., Boyd, K.M., Templeton, A.A., and Potter, B. Research ethical committees in Scotland. *Br. med. J.,* **282,** 718–20 (1981).
40. Allen, P.A., Waters, W.E., and McGreen, A.M. Research ethical committees in 1981. *Jnl R. Coll. Physicians Lond.* **17,** 96–8 (1983).
41. —— and —— Development of an ethical committee and its effect on research design. *Lancet* **i,** 1233–6 (1982).
42. Ethical committee, University College Hospital. Experience at a clinical research ethical review committee. *Br. med. J.* **283,** 1312–14 (1981).
43. Denham, M.J., Foster, A., and Tyrrell, D.A.J. Work of a district ethical committee. *Br. med. J.* **2,** 1042-5 (1979).
44. Working group in current medical/ethical problems, Northern Regional Health Authority. Applications for ethical approval. *Lancet* **i,** 87-9 (1978).
45. O'Brien, M. Clinical research and its ethical control in Durham between 1974 and 1979. *Public Health (London)* **94,** 288–93 (1980).
46. Council of the British Medical Association. Local ethical committees. *Br. med. J.* **282,** 1010 (1981).
47. British Medical Association, Central Ethical Committee. *Local ethical research committees.* B.M.A. London (1984).
48. Royal College of Physicians. *Guidelines on the practice of ethics committees in medical research.* RCP, London (1984).
49. Ryan, M.K. General organization of the IRB. In *Human subjects research: a handbook for institutional review boards* (eds. R.A. Greenwald, M.K. Ryan, and J.E. Mulvihill) pp.29–38. Plenum, New York (1982).
50. O'Brien, M. and Mahadevan, S. A system for the ethical control of clinical research. *Public Health (London)* **94,** 219–222 (1980).
51. Gray, B.H., Cooke, R.A., and Tannenbaum, A.S. Research involving human subjects. *Science* **201,** 1094–101 (1978).
52. Altman, D.G. Statistics and ethics in medical research. In *Statistics in practice* (eds. S.M. Gore and D.G. Altman) pp1–24. British Medical Association, London (1982).

53. Tannenbaum, A.S. and Cooke, R.A. Research involving children. In *Appendix to report and recommendations: Research involving children* (National Commission for the Protection of Human Subjects of Biomedical and Behavioral Research). DHEW (77-0005), Washington DC (1977).
54. Greenwald, R.A. Informed consent. In *Human subjects research: a handbook for institutional review boards* (eds. R.A. Greenwald, M.K. Ryan, and J.E. Mulvihill) pp.79–90. Plenum, New York (1982).
55. British Paediatric Association. Guidelines to aid ethical committees considering research involving children. *Archs Dis. Childh.* **55,** 75–7 (1980).
56. Dunstan, G.R. and Seller, M.J. (eds.) *Consent in medicine,* pp.57-84. King Edward's Hospital Fund for London, London (1983).
57. Heath, E.J. The IRB's monitoring function: four concepts of monitoring. *IRB: a review of human subjects research* **1**(5), 1–3 and 12 (1979).

9

The conduct of research

Various aspects of research on children have been considered in earlier chapters. In the Introduction, controls on research were discussed, as was the somewhat confusing state of current guidelines for research on children. The second chapter essayed some definitions of terms that have been used in this report, and in particular the distinction between therapeutic and non-therapeutic research. Subsequent chapters examined the scope of, and need for, research on children, and the philosophical and legal constraints within which it should be undertaken. Chapter 5 indicated the limitations, with our present knowledge, of risk assessment, while suggesting the likelihood, in the future, of accurate risk/benefit analysis being of great importance in the ethical assessment of research projects. The two preceding chapters have discussed the extent to which children themselves might be involved in the process of giving informed consent to research procedures, and some of the ways in which research ethics committees assess research proposals. The purpose of this chapter is to consider more closely some of the practical aspects of research on children that have been suggested by the previous chapters. It is proposed to examine the progress of a research project from the first bright idea to publication.

If an investigator or a clinician has a bright idea which, after due reflection, still seems to be worth further examination, there are essentially two ways in which he may try to find out whether it is likely to benefit children. Either he may set up a research project to investigate the questions posed by his bright idea, or the idea may lead him directly to a new or variant treatment – an innovative therapy – which he decides to test in an unsystematic manner. In either case, unless the bright idea occurs to him during a medical or surgical emergency that he is treating, there are certain preliminaries to be undertaken. One that is common to both innovative therapy and a research project is the duty on the investigator to acquaint himself thoroughly with the literature already available in his field of enquiry. With the advent in most large libraries of computer facilities for searching the literature such a duty is relatively easy to fulfil nowadays. Should the British Paediatric Association set up the register of paediatric research in progress that has been suggested,[1] it will be possible for an investigator to find out not only whether his idea has been examined in a previous published report, but also whether any work is in progress, at least in Great Britain. Another, recently developed, source of such information is the Medical Research Directory;[2] neither resource, however, is likely to prevent duplication of research in progress in other countries.

Planning a research project

If the investigator decides to proceed by means of a research project, there is much to be done as well as a literature search before he could contemplate approaching either a research ethics committee or a funding body with his proposal. There are the questions to be asked that were mentioned in Chapter 5:

(i) Is the right question being asked?
(ii) Is this project the best way to answer it?
(iii) If the project should provide an answer, will it be worth knowing?

Question (ii) involves several considerations, such as whether relevant experiments on animals or tissues have already been carried out. If all the information has been obtained that can be from animal experiments and tissues, then one must ask whether the research could not be carried out on adult humans, rather than on children. It is at this stage that an investigator should be preparing a risk/benefit analysis as discussed in Chapter 5. He should be considering whether his proposed research methods involve interventions of as low a level of risk and upset as possible. Even for such a routine procedure, for instance, as a heel-prick to obtain a blood sample from an infant, there are more and less painful ways of carrying out the procedure. He should be aware that a mechanical device, the Autolet, is considerably less painful when used to obtain blood than a heel-prick performed by hand.[3] At this stage also the investigator should decide whether his proposed research would benefit from economic analysis. There is a growing body of opinion which suggests that economic analysis should be incorporated as a part of most clinical trials so as to give an indication of the relative costs of the regimens being assessed. The place of such analysis has been reviewed by Drummond and Stoddart.[4] The purpose of the questions (i)–(iii) above is to try to ensure that the research project should be scientifically sound and capable of providing a significant result. There are differing views as to whether questions of scientific merit should be considered also by a research ethics committee, and these are discussed elsewhere.

Another important element in many research projects nowadays is the statistical analysis that is to be employed. The use of appropriate statistical methods allows a researcher to conclude a project when the minimum number of research subjects has been used to produce a result that is significant both statistically and clinically. If one may produce a significant result by performing a procedure on a small number of children, it is obviously preferable to end the project then, rather than to continue until an arbitrarily larger number of children have been involved. A study by Morton and Lawande,[5] for instance, was designed to determine whether supra-pubic aspiration of urine could be carried out safely and successfully in children aged 10 years and below, attending the outpatients department of a Nigerian teaching hospital. 287 supra-pubic aspirations were carried out, but in only 51 cases were midstream specimens of urine collected from patients who had also had supra-pubic aspiration. In all 51 cases both specimens of urine gave similar results, with no false positive or false negative results. On the basis of these 51 double results the authors conclude that a single midstream specimen of urine would give a reliable indication of a urinary tract infection provided the specimen was handled correctly. One wonders, however, why it was necessary to perform 287 supra-pubic aspirations, which involve the insertion of a needle through the lower abdominal wall directly into the bladder. It was possible to show a first-time success rate of 91 per cent, which was directly comparable to previous reports. In 5 cases, bowel contents rather than urine were obtained by accident: four of these children could be followed up and they developed no complications. Only 51 aspirations were needed for comparison with midstream specimens of urine, and hardly any more than that would have been needed to show that it was a relatively straightforward, if invasive, procedure. On the other hand, 287 aspirations would not be enough to establish the safety of the procedure: it might be, for instance, that one in twenty of the children whose bowels were entered went on to develop peritonitis. That would give a risk of a major complication of about one in a thousand, which would not be likely to be picked up in this study. It illustrates the need to decide the purpose, or end-point, of a study, and then to calculate statistically the number of subjects to include in the study in order to reach that end-point.

Controlled trials

Some research projects will be designed as randomized controlled trials: these are now regarded as the principal means of assessing the efficacy of a new therapy, or of comparing a new therapy with an existing one. The basis of such a trial is that each subject is allocated at random either to a 'control' group which is treated with a placebo or with the existing therapy, or else to a treatment group which is treated with the new therapy. (See Chapter 2, pp.31–3, for further discussion of controls). There has been considerable discussion recently of the ethics of such trials, but only a brief summary of the debate will be offered here.

Randomized trials came to public attention as a result of an inquest held on an elderly widow who had died in September, 1981 from bone-marrow depression induced by fluorouracil.[6] She had been given fluorouracil without her knowledge or consent during a controlled trial of chemotherapy following resection of cancer of the large bowel. It became evident at the inquest that several local research ethics committees had approved the enrolment of subjects into this trial without the subjects' informed consents being obtained at any stage. Subsequently, Brewin[7] argued that the subject's informed consent was not needed in such trials, since two treatment options were being compared; in the course of normal treatment doctors had to decide between different treatment possibilities and usually did so without informing their patients of all the pros and cons of each possibility. Patients trusted the doctor to come to the best decision for them. His argument, however, is based on some special pleading: that, since 'research', according to him, has no precise definition, one cannot use the word to describe randomized treatment – as he chooses to call randomized controlled trials of treatment. It is more generally accepted, however, that such trials are indeed a part of research, because there would be no point in randomizing treatment unless as part of a carefully recorded study. His argument also depends on the idea that a doctor does not need to give a patient nearly so much information when asking for consent to treatment as when seeking consent to a research procedure: such an approach is probably unacceptably paternalistic to many patients nowadays.

Randomized controlled trials, in which a clinician or researcher abdicates his responsibility to offer the best possible treatment to his patients, can only be ethical if he is unable to choose between the efficacies of the treatments to be given at random. If he wishes to compare a new drug with a placebo he must do so because he is genuinely uncertain that the drug will be of benefit, and there is no accepted treatment for the condition for which the drug is being tested. When there is already an accepted best treatment, then any new drug must be compared with it. It is possible, however, to use such trials in inappropriate circumstances, some of which have been discussed by Hofmann.[8] An example of the misuse of the controlled trial, when a placebo was used unethically in a trial comparing several drugs already known to be effective against schistosomiasis, may be found in a paper by Pugh and Teesdale.[9] The precise purpose of the trial is not stated: the only indication is that 'the trial was conducted as a preliminary to studies of mass treatment in *Schistosoma haematobium* infections'. In Malawi, 433 primary school children were stratified into four groups according to age (overall 5–18 years) and further stratified according to the degree of schistosomal infestation as assessed by the number of ova excreted in their urine. They were then allocated at random either to one of the three treatment groups or to one of two control groups, in each case receiving a single oral dose. The first group received praziquantel, a highly effective and safe drug, but one which is five times more expensive than the preparation received by the second group, a combination of metrifonate and niridazole. This combination is known to have a lower efficacy than praziquantel, as is metrifonate by itself, which was received by the third treatment group; metrifonate, however, costs only one-eighteenth as much per dose as praziquantel. The first control group was given a dose of niridazole alone 'since it was a component of the combined regimen, and it is normally given alone for at least five days to be effective'. The second control group was given a placebo – in fact, ascorbic acid, vitamin C.

The authors used two control groups because 'the level of transmission (of the parasitic fluke) could have influenced the chemotherapeutic response of the treated subjects who remained in contact
with potentially contaminated water.' They refer to a paper by
McMahon[10] in justification: he makes the point that not only does
the level of transmission vary according to the season, but that the
level of excretion of ova in the urine may decrease for reasons not
related to chemotherapy. He therefore makes a strong recommendation for the use of control groups in trials of anti-
schistosomal drugs in order to avoid misleading conclusions as to
drug efficacy. His arguments appear irrelevant in the context of
Pugh and Teesdale's trial, however. So far as one may gather from
their report, the purpose of the trial seems not to have been to
establish that the drugs used were effective since that was already
known; the purpose was to compare their efficacies in a particular
group of children treated at the same time. Moreover, McMahon's
paper provides no support at all for the use of two control groups.
It would appear that the authors had some inkling of the impro-
priety of the trial since they comment: 'In accordance with local
ethical guidelines the placebo group (given vitamin C) consisted
only of children with light or moderate infections before treatment.' Nevertheless, at the three-month follow-up, 25 per cent of
the placebo group required treatment for a heavy infection, compared with 46.3 per cent of the first control group (given niridazole
alone), and 0 per cent, 0 per cent, and 4.3 per cent of the three
treatment groups. The trial illustrates the extreme care that is
needed in deciding what treatments may be compared in a trial and
whether it is necessary to have a placebo group.

Schafer has reviewed[11] the ethical problems of randomized clinical trials, commenting, *inter alia*, on the conflict of obligations of
the physician to his patient or to the furtherance of medical knowledge (the role conflict discussed in Chapter 3) and on the need to
sacrifice individualized treatment. He also considers the problem
of whether or not a physician should admit to a preference for one
of the alternative treatments if he has such a preference, and the
difficulties of obtaining informed consent if a patient is told that his
treatment will be decided at random. Lockwood considers there to
be an ethical problem in the non-treatment of patients who act as
controls in controlled trials.[12] His argument is based on cases such
as that given in Chapter 3 in which the action of high levels of inspired oxygen in producing blindness in premature infants was

investigated; before that trial was started there was already considerable evidence suggesting a link between high levels of oxygen and blindness. Lockwood seeks to generalize from such exceptional examples to the idea that researchers will usually feel that one of the treatments to be tested is better than the other, or that the single treatment to be tested is better than a placebo, thus making the continuation of the trial unethical. It is, however, very commonly the case that doctors cannot objectively distinguish the efficacies of the two options before a controlled trial: provided that the statistical design of the trial allows the earliest possible recognition of a significant difference, and provided that doctors act on this information, Lockwood's argument fails. The relationship between the statistical design of trials and their ethical status has been examined in more depth by Clayton[13] and by Altman.[14]

An alternative design for randomized clinical trials has also been proposed by Zelen.[15] He suggests that patients be allocated at random either to receive the best standard treatment or to be in a second group. The second group are asked whether they will accept the new treatment. In analysing the results, all those in the second group, regardless of the treatment they actually received, are compared with those in the first group, who just received the best standard treatment. Such a scheme could not be used when a 'double-blind' trial is essential, i.e. a trial in which neither the researcher nor the patient knows which treatment the patient is receiving. It is, in fact, the main advantage of Zelen's proposed design for trials that the patient does know whether he is receiving the new, experimental treatment, and is not expected to give his consent to a random choice of treatment. The statistical disadvantage of the design is that any effects of the new treatment may be 'diluted' by those in the second group who refused the new treatment, so that a larger number of patients will be needed in the trial to obtain significant results.

Selection of subjects

The ethical problems of clinical trials have been,[16–19] and will continue to be, extensively debated elsewhere. It is intended here only to give a brief introduction to some of the relevant literature. Nor is it possible to discuss more than a very few of the elements in the scientific design of a trial, since every research project will have design features that are individual to itself. It is important, however, to consider some of the problems of selection of subjects for projects. Most doctors who do research work in hospitals, and therefore have easiest access to children who are either already in the wards or maternity unit nursery, or who attend regularly as out-patients. Mention has already been made of the increased emotional strains that may exist in children with chronic illnesses and in their families. If the design of the research project will require children to remain longer in wards, to have more stays as in-patients, or to attend more often as out-patients, it is important that the investigator be aware of the family strain or even disruption that may be caused and try to reduce the chances both of present distress and future emotional disturbance.

The other main problem with the use of children who are already in hospital or an institution is that they may be used in research of little or no relevance to their own condition, just because they are there and available. This seems to be a distinct possibility in some neonatal nurseries, and perhaps particularly in those in which informed parental consent to research procedures is often not sought. Another example given to the working group involved a bone-marrow transplant programme. The nurses felt that some investigators not directly involved in the programme had realized that a captive group of research subjects was available for projects that were not related to their original illness. A further group of children who are readily available to investigators are mentally retarded or otherwise handicapped children living permanently in institutions.

An example of the sort of project that may be carried out is a study of the use of clindamycin in the treatment of chronic recurrent suppurative otitis media in children. This was in fact carried out in the United States, but reported[20] in a British journal, with no mention of consent being obtained from the parents or guardians of the children involved, or of Institutional Review Board approval having been obtained, although it might have been. In this study, 28 mentally retarded residents of a Californian 'hospital facility', aged from 13 months to 9 years and 10 months, had acute middle-ear infections. They were described as having 'chronic recurrent suppurative otitis media', yet all had intact ear-drums, through which a needle was passed – a process called tympanocentesis – to obtain a sample of pus from the middle ear. All were then treated with clindamycin, an antibiotic which the manufacturer's own literature says should only be used in serious infections, because of the substantial risk of a serious, and in some cases life-threatening, side-effect, known as pseudo-membranous colitis. They were given a dose of 30 to 40 mg/kg per day, i.e. approximately double the British National Formulary recommendation[21] of 12 to 24 mg/kg/day or a standard paediatric textbook's recommendation[22] of 10 to 25 mg/kg/day, and the course of treatment lasted 17 days on average. Fortunately, no episodes of colitis ensued. The results of the bacteriological studies confirmed the presence of anaerobic organisms in a majority of the children's ears, a finding which other studies have produced over a period of about 80 years. Just over half the infections (16/28) cleared up on treatment, although in 7 of those cases gentamicin had been added to the treatment regime.

There are obviously many criticisms that may be made of this study. Consent would not have been available from the children, and it is not stated that it was obtained from their parents or guardians. The diagnoses appear in doubt since it is highly unusual to talk of an acute exacerbation of chronic recurrent suppurative otitis media when the eardrums remain intact. An antibiotic with a well-recognized risk of a serious side-effect was used at double the normal dosage and for at least twice as long as usual, when other antibiotics effective against anaerobic organisms were available. It seems difficult to accept that such a project would have received ethics committee approval had it been proposed for the ear, nose, and throat department of a general hospital. One is left with the perhaps unjustified suspicion that the project happened only because a captive group of retarded children was available. It is, in passing, worrying that the report of such a project can still be published in a British journal. There is not space to discuss here the continuing controversy as to whether reports of projects that may have been conducted in an unethical manner should or should not be published; readers wishing to pursue the question are referred to an excellent review by DeBakey.[23]

A further problem in the selection of children for projects arises when children of a particular social or ethnic group are to be included. The introductory statement to one survey of schoolchildren, as reported[24] in the *British Medical Journal*, could readily have caused offence: 'To assess whether immigrant children from tropical and subtropical countries have transmissible infections and infestations that might constitute a health hazard to native Scottish children we designed a survey to compare health and nutrition in Asian, African and Chinese children with those in Scottish children of similar social background.' It is interesting that the only intestinal parasite that was at all common was giardia lamblia, the highest incidence being in the Scottish children. The Inner London Education Authority has taken note of the possible discrimination in this sort of selection in its statement *Policy on external research applications*:[25] 'most schools are reluctant to allow researchers to test only selected pupils in a class (e.g. those of a particular ethnic or social group). Researchers may be obliged to test whole classes and extract the results of pupils in whom they are interested afterwards.'

A final consideration in the selection of children for a project is financial. A study[26] in Birmingham examined the financial consequences to fifty-nine families of the treatment of cancer in children referred to a regional oncology centre. 'During the first, in-patient, week of treatment the sum of income lost plus additional expenditure exceeded 50% of total income in over 45% of families. During a subsequent week of out-patient treatment, loss of income plus additional expenditure amounted to more than 20% of income in over half the families'. A survey[27] of four special care baby units carried out in the autumn of 1980 showed a wide variation in the total travelling costs expended by parents on visiting their infants. The costs ranged from £1 to £518, with means of £41 and £123 respectively for parents of inborn and outborn infants travelling by car, and £30 and £46 respectively for parents using public transport. The financial implications of any research project that requires additional attendances by a child, or additional time spent as an in-patient, should be recognized, and appropriate expenses paid. It is important, however, that any payments should be only to cover expenses or loss of income, and should not be large enough to act as an inducement to parents to enter their children into a research project. There have been two recent examples of substantial payments to research subjects; in one case only unemployed people were to be used as subjects; in the other, medical students were paid sums running into hundreds of pounds to take part in drug research carried out by a private research organization. While it is not certain that such payments to adults act as inducements, or draw into question the voluntary nature of any consent given to a research procedure, it is certainly true that it would be unethical to induce parents to offer their children as research subjects by paying them any substantial reward. There are occasions, however, when a small present to the children involved may be appropriate. In a study of the value of determining tooth lead-levels, children who gave a tooth were given a badge which indicated that they had done so: a psychologist involved in the study commented that the badges had given a considerable boost to the self-esteem of the child subjects.

One consequence of research projects that may receive inadequate attention during the planning stage is the extra work that may be created for nurses, in particular, but also for other staff such as medical records officers. This is primarily a problem of resource allocation: any project that does create extra work should include provision for employing extra staff adequate to cope with the extra work. An example given to the working group was that of 24-hour urine collections, used for the measurement of the rate of excretion of a large number of substances. Collections over 24 hours in small children can be very difficult to complete: the collecting bags that are stuck over their genitalia may leak, become contaminated by faeces, or be pulled off by the children. It might sometimes take five days to complete a satisfactory collection, and it requires considerable honesty and self-control from the nurses to start again when something goes wrong. If that sort of workload for research purposes is added to the routine ward work, it could lead to a decrease in the level of care provided for other patients, that would in most circumstances represent an unacceptable consequence of a research project.

By this stage of planning, an investigator is just about ready to submit his bright idea as a research project to funding bodies and a research ethics committee. Before doing so, he would be wise to check that his motives for undertaking the project do include a desire to gain new knowledge or to improve some aspect of children's health. In Chapter 3 the incentive for doctors to improve their career prospects by undertaking research was mentioned. Margaret Mead has discussed[28] the dangers of research that is inspired by rivalry with other investigators, or that is the uncritical pursuit of a fashionable ideal. She comments: 'Anthropological research does not have subjects. We work with informants in an atmosphere of trust and mutual respect', and stresses the 'possibility of regarding human subjects as participants in a collective enterprise'. This represents an important emphasis that can be summed up by the substitution of 'with' for 'on' in the phrase 'research on children' – which, incidentally, was written into the title of the working group which produced this report. This tends to suggest that research is carried out on objects, rather than the conventional 'research subject'. It is perhaps a minor semantic point, but promotion of the notion that research is 'with children', or 'with human subjects', rather than 'on' them, might serve to remind investigators that research should be a partnership. The responsibility for what is done to a research subject must always rest ultimately with the investigator, rather than with a research ethics committee or any other institution; the concept of research as a partnership would serve to promote awareness of this responsibility.

Submission of research proposals to research ethics committees

The potential investigator is now ready to submit his proposal for research with some children to his local research ethics committee. He may wonder whether it is really necessary to do so; after all, he may say, it was perfectly easy to answer the questions that an investigator should be asked (p.196): the proposed research is designed to help children. He may also be aware that his local research ethics committee is one of the 12 per cent (according to the survey in Chapter 8) that do not regard it as obligatory for all research proposals to be submitted to the committee for approval. It would be very simple, and perfectly legal, to get on with the research, possibly adding to the number of chairmen of research ethics committees (already 11 per cent) who are aware of research taking place within their 'jurisdiction' for which ethics committee approval had not been sought.

The most likely reason in practice why an investigator, already sure of the ethical propriety of his project, will nevertheless submit his proposal to a research ethics committee is money. The great majority of organizations that provide funds for medical research insist that anyone applying for money to carry out a particular project should already have ethics committee approval for the project. If his local ethics committee is one of those remarkable ones that also allocate, or make recommendations for the allocation of, research funds, then he will have an added incentive to submit his proposal. There are, however, some important reasons in principle, as well as in practice, why research proposals should be submitted to ethics committees.

The history of the establishment of research ethics committees was outlined in Chapter 8. Public attention had been drawn to the fact that some clinical research investigators appeared to exploit, to put in hazard, or to violate, some research subjects. This was perhaps an inevitable consequence of there being no specific controls on research on human beings, whereas research on animals had been controlled ever since the passing of the Cruelty to Animals Act 1876. One might have hoped that informed peer review would provide adequate control of clinical research activities, but sadly there is little evidence of any form of peer review being readily acceptable to British doctors. The working group was told of several attempts to set up regular meetings to review mortality and morbidity in various units. In a paediatric surgical unit the majority of surgeons had been reluctant to go to meetings with their colleagues to discuss implications of their operations. In a maternity hospital, the majority of cases discussed at the monthly perinatal morbidity meetings came from one unit: the consultant in charge of that unit attended the meetings regularly, yet he never changed his practice, but continued to make the same errors of judgement. It has been suggested that the most effective form of peer review in clinical research is the knowledge that unethical research will not be published. Yet almost every example of published research given in this report has been published in a British journal, even though many of the investigations were actually carried out abroad; there are several amongst them that can only be regarded as unethical.

The vast majority of clinical investigators want to undertake research in an ethical manner and succeed in doing so. But the evidence of Beecher[29] and Pappworth,[30] and of other sporadic examples more recently, has caused the public to be less trusting of researchers than in the past. Thus some sort of control on research became essential: the absence of any tradition of successful informal peer review of clinical or research activities made it inevitable that the more formal system of research ethics committees would be established. It is a system that causes investigators varying degrees of displeasure that tend to be inversely related to the speed, and sometimes directly related to the thoroughness, with which particular committees function. Yet the committees may have much to offer the investigator. They have built up bodies of expertise that can help investigators to plan their projects better, whether by examining some of the elements of planning a project discussed earlier in this chapter, or by discussing the ways in which information is to be given to parents and children and their consent gained. Should anything go wrong during the course of clinical research, a researcher is likely to be in a better position in the event of litigation if he has had ethics committee approval than in its absence, even though such approval is not yet legally mandatory. The general acceptance of research ethics committees, and their promotion by the Royal College of Physicians, the DHSS, and the British Medical Association, mean that an investigator who does not submit a research proposal for ethics committee approval is increasingly likely to find himself in a difficult position. This was illustrated by the public outcry in 1983[31] when it was discovered that a registrar at a London teaching hospital was carrying out trials of calcium and vitamin D supplementation in pregnant Asian women. The trial was of questionable safety, had not been submitted to the local research ethics committee, and was only stopped when other junior staff – not the consultant in charge – complained.

Projects involving minor procedures

There are, nevertheless, doubts and confusion among investigators as to whether all research projects should be submitted for ethics committee approval. One area of uncertainty concerns the level at which the degree of intervention involved in a procedure is so minor that ethics committee approval becomes superfluous. Several examples were given to the working group of research procedures that involved such minor interventions that opinion is divided as to whether they need assessment by a research ethics committee.

It is a relatively common procedure, as for instance in a project designed to establish a normal paediatric range for the level of plasma amylase,[32] to take a couple of extra millilitres of blood for a research purpose during the course of a venepuncture necessary to the routine management of the patient/subject. A very competent ward sister was interested in replacing mercury thermometers on her children's ward by electronic thermometers; before doing so, she wished to compare for herself the accuracies of the new and old thermometers and to see whether there were any practical problems in the use of the new thermometers. For two weeks, therefore, every child in her ward had its temperature measurements performed in duplicate, which was obviously not a standard ward procedure. A psychologist administered a picture memory test to children waiting to be seen in an ENT outpatients department, as part of a pilot study to test its efficacy. She thought one member of the working group to be mad when he asked whether she had considered that her project should perhaps have been submitted to the local research ethics committee for approval. In research into the treatment of eczema, an objective assessment of its severity is provided by measuring limb movement; a proposal to do so by asking children to wear modified self-winding watches was delayed for months by the wait for ethics committee approval. In studying zinc deficiency, zinc levels had been measured regularly on specimens of blood: ethics committee approval was required in order to use a method of measuring zinc levels on a few hairs.

To suggest that such projects require ethics committee approval, as indeed was the case in the latter two, might at first sight seem excessively officious. Discussion of a further example by the working group, however, suggested that even apparently simple research projects might have more serious implications such as should be considered by an ethics committee.

It is quite common for medical students to be encouraged to undertake small research projects: because of the full teaching programmes already arranged, such projects are often arranged and carried out over a period of a few months only. One such project, at a London teaching hospital, was for two students to record electrocardiograms (ECGs) from children admitted routinely for tonsillectomy and adenoidectomy. It is known that about 4 per cent of such children have sufficient tonsillar and adenoidal enlargement to cause a degree of respiratory obstruction that results in heart strain. Such heart strain can be demonstrated on an ECG, and may increase the operative risk for the child, and give rise to long-term heart problems. The ECGs were obtained by the students whenever they had time, regardless of whether the parents were present. Parental consent was not obtained, the recording of an ECG being a completely routine part of the investigation of children with a variety of conditions, although not being a routine part of the pre-operative assessment of such children. The project was non-invasive, potentially therapeutic, research of negligible risk, was descriptive in that there was no control group, and was intended to replicate results previously obtained elsewhere. The primary intent was to provide a training exercise for the two students, but there was an intent also to add to knowledge in this field; there was even a third intent, that the project might identify those children who were at risk because of heart strain. Submission of the project to the local research ethics committee would have so delayed it as to make it impossible for the students to carry out.

One member of this working group, also a member of a research ethics committee, thought that the project should have been submitted for ethics committee approval: it was likely that the committee would have insisted on the obtaining of parental consent, and that it would have insisted on adequate supervision of the students by a doctor. The latter might have been of considerable benefit to the children: the students were not trusted to read the ECGs, so that information that might be of value to the operating team was generally not available to them before the operation; closer supervision could have led to competent assessment of the ECGs pre-operatively. Another member of the working group pointed out that a substantial proportion of the parents of any children admitted to hospital feared that their children had a more serious illness, such as cancer, than they had been told; an unexplained procedure such as recording an ECG could increase rather than allay such fears. While the procedure was physically harmless, it could upset small children, particularly if undertaken in the absence of their parents.

Thus, the project had implications that were not adequately taken into consideration by the rather casual approach adopted in order to let the students complete the project. It is of interest that student projects elsewhere have to be submitted to the local ethics committee: this is a useful practice, since medical students need to be encouraged to develop ethical awareness as well as to learn about research methods. Figures provided by Allen and Waters[33] show that just over half the submissions to the ethics committee for Southampton and South-west Hampshire during a five-year period, 1977–81, were made by fourth-year medical students at Southampton University.

There is no obvious answer to the question of which projects involving minor procedures should be submitted to a research ethics committee and which need not be. In any project requiring invasive procedures, the child's physical integrity is the paramount concern, and ethics committee approval should be mandatory. On the other hand, if the only invasion is of the subject's privacy, such as in observational studies that require no interaction, then parental consent by itself should be adequate to allow the researcher to proceed. Thus, the taking of additional blood, even during a routine procedure, should be assessed by an ethics committee.

The other projects, such as recording ECGs or limb movement, or taking a few hairs, remain in a grey area. It is suggested that they should all be submitted to a research ethics committee. The investigator will have nothing to lose, and may indeed gain by the committee's consideration of some of the implications, as suggested in the discussion above of the student project for ECG recording. His main objection to submitting his proposal will probably be that the committee will cause unnecessary – in his view – delay in his project. This problem was discussed in Chapter 8, in which it was suggested that the solution is to make much greater use of expedited review, by the chairman of the ethics committee in particular.

New instruments

Another area of uncertainty as to whether a submission to a research ethics committee is required concerns the introduction of new instruments. In some instances it is evident that such a submission would be superfluous. If a doctor has been routinely examining children's stomachs with a gastroscope of 8 mm external diameter, there could be no possible argument against his using a new instrument that was similar in all respects other than that its external diameter was only 6.5 mm. It is self-evident that the new instrument would be easier to pass, and would probably cause the children on whom it was used less discomfort.

The introduction of new instruments sometimes makes new procedures possible, and in these cases it may be more difficult to suggest that ethics committee approval is not needed. In recent years, fibreoptic technology has made possible total colonoscopy in children. A series of 123 such procedures was reported in 1982 by Williams *et al.*;[34] they comment that 97 per cent were 'performed with sedation only'. One is left to assume that the remaining 3 per cent required anaesthesia. The same group have recently reported[35] their experience of using a very flexible paediatric colonoscope to perform a more limited examination of the rectum and sigmoid colon. Previously, such examination in children required the passage of a rigid instrument under general anaesthetic. The report states: 'Fibreoptic procto-sigmoidoscopy was added without formality to the routine outpatient physical examination. No prior bowel preparation was given and no sedation was used before, during or after the procedure.' The procedure was carried out on 21 children aged 4 to 15 years.

It appears that this was a new procedure in that previously sedation and bowel preparation had always been given before the passage of a colonoscope. It was not stated either that parental consent or research ethics committee approval had been obtained, although they may have been. The expression 'without formality' to describe the introduction of the procedure suggests that it was intended that parents and children should accept the procedure as routine. At all events, such a procedure seems to be so far removed from routine practice that research ethics committee approval should have been sought for it. A clear indication of appropriate ethical concern is, however, provided in the description of the first use of nuclear magnetic resonance imaging of children's brains by Levene *et al.*[36] Experience in adults had shown several features of such imaging that might be of particular benefit in paediatric practice. Research ethics committee approval was obtained, as was informed parental consent, and the procedure was performed on 4 normal children and 18 children thought to have various cerebral pathologies.

Innovative therapy

It was suggested at the beginning of this chapter that an investigator having a bright idea might decide to proceed either by way of a research project or by trying out an innovative therapy in a haphazard fashion. There are at present no formal controls on innovative therapy, a lack which can sometimes lead to a major problem. Essentially, a doctor may try out any new idea he likes, so long as he does it in a haphazard way; if he wants to be properly scientific about it, and set up a systematic study, that is called research, and automatically becomes subject to a number of controls. Some investigators now believe that patients are often at greater risk from innovative therapies, that have not been subject either to informal peer review or to formal ethics committee assessment, than from research projects that are non-therapeutic in intention. An example of such a hazard – in adults rather than children – is given by a new technique designed to reopen blocked coronary arteries, thus obviating the need for coronary bypass surgery. A balloon device is passed into an artery and advanced into the blocked coronary artery in order to perform a procedure known as transluminal coronary angioplasty. In the early days of this procedure, various operators tried it out in small uncontrolled series to which a lot of publicity was then given. Had a drug been used to achieve the same effect, however, there would have been a trial procedure lasting several years with very tight controls.

The example given above of an innovative therapy was of a new surgical technique: it does indeed appear to be advances in surgical technique that constitute most examples of uncontrolled innovative therapy. Where possible new techniques are tested on animals and then on adults before trying them out on children. Reports of paediatric surgery studies are frequently of comparisons between surgical techniques: that such comparisons are necessary is perhaps indicated by information given to the working group that over 150 surgical techniques have been described for the correction of hypospadias alone. A typical paper might compare three different techniques for the relief of Hirschsprung's disease: since all three techniques are already accepted it is unlikely that the surgeon would request research ethics committee approval, or obtain parental consent for a research procedure rather than just for a routine operation. Such an example does indicate, however, that there can be research projects in paediatric surgery as well as the use of innovative therapies: another example shows that such trials may have a danger that is not usually met in comparative trials of drugs. The working group was told of a proposed trial which involved comparing two techniques for the surgical treatment of hypertrophic pyloric stenosis, a relatively common condition in infants, in which the outflow from the stomach is blocked. The classical operation, introduced in 1912, is Ramstedt's procedure; this was to be compared with endoscopic balloon disruption, in which an endoscope is passed through the stomach into the pylorus, or outflow; the tumour was then to be disrupted by inflating a balloon lying within it. This method had been attempted many years previously and had been abandoned following the near perfect results obtained by the Ramstedt procedure. The proposed trial was addressed to answering the wrong question: it should have been directed to examining why the results of the Ramstedt operation in the unit planning the trial were so poor rather than to proposing an alternative procedure. It also illustrates one difficulty of comparative surgical trials: that there may be much less consistency in the efficacy of a certain surgical procedure than one would expect were a particular drug to be used in various trials.

Most innovations in paediatric surgery are minor modifications to, or improvements in, surgical technique, some of which will only suggest themselves to the operator during the course of an operation. The innovations such as that referred to in Chapter 2, when a new surgical correction for transposition of the great arteries was introduced with a startling increase in mortality, are fortunately uncommon. Surgeons may frequently, however, try out an idea, and perhaps complete a series of forty or fifty operations: their results may show no benefit from the innovation or even actual harm, in which case the results are unlikely ever to see the light of day, since editors do not usually publish poor or failed research. Just as, therefore, occasional disasters in more formal research led to a demand for the control provided by research ethics committees, so too it would be valuable to develop a system for the supervision of innovative therapy. Yet the very nature of the majority of innovations makes such a proposal likely to be impractical. It is essential that surgeons and others be allowed some degree of freedom in developing innovations. Indeed, there is some evidence that the law protects just such a freedom: the law governing compensation for injuries to unborn children[37] states that a doctor should not be liable for negligence just because he goes beyond the limits of normal or accepted practice. On the other hand, it might still be held, in some circumstances, that a surgeon had acted negligently if he had failed to inform a patient that a new technique was to be used.

One needs to consider what sort of limit could be placed on the doctors' and surgeons' freedom to introduce innovations, so as to protect patients from unnecessary risks while not curtailing the freedom excessively. It would obviously be impossible to demand that every innovation be subject to some sort of peer review before it was first carried out: such a rule would eliminate the instantaneous, and often very useful, ideas that arise during an operation or an emergency. On the other hand, it might be reasonable to adopt a rule of thumb that after some innovation had been tried, say, five times it should become subject to peer review, probably by a research ethics committee. If the innovation had been a failure every time, such a rule might prevent an innovator from carrying on with it endlessly, in the hope that it might eventually work. If, however, the innovation showed some promise after it had been tried five times, the need to submit a more formal proposal to a research ethics committee would ensure that an objective assessment of its value would be undertaken at the earliest possible time. Such a scheme would be impossible to monitor, and would rely totally on the willingness of doctors and surgeons to submit themselves to such review of their innovative therapies. The advantages, however, in terms of protecting the public, and ensuring quicker and more objective assessment of innovations, are such that it is to be hoped that such a rule of thumb might soon be adopted.

The practice of research

The investigator has now submitted his bright idea to a research ethics committee, either as a research project *ab initio* or perhaps after he has tried out his innovative therapy just a few times. The committee has considered the proposal and its various implications in the manner suggested in the previous chapter, and the researcher has been pleasantly surprised by the rapidity of the committee's decision. He has (lucky fellow) had no difficulty in securing funds for the research, and is now ready to invade the children's ward to find suitable subjects for his project. There is, however, one important thing to be done first: to inform the other staff on the ward of his intentions. There are two main reasons for doing so: first, it is highly likely that some degree of help will be needed from the staff – whether it be simply to find children for him, or actually to help in research procedures such as urine collection; secondly, it is inevitable that the staff will be asked about what the researcher is doing. There is a third reason also: nurses sometimes complain that they do not know whether a research project has been approved by the research ethics committee.

Nurses do not normally play an important part in gaining consent from parents for procedures on their children, whether they be routine therapy or research. Invariably, however, on a children's ward the nurses are asked detailed questions by parents, not only about the physical procedures to be performed on their children, but also about risks and prognoses. It is well known that less than half the medical information given to patients or parents in an interview is retained by them once the interview is finished. The usual recourse of parents is to ask anyone else available, whether that person be nurse, auxiliary, play leader, ward cleaner, or, most commonly, another parent. It is therefore essential that the nurses at least, and perhaps also other staff, should be given adequate information about the project so that they can answer parents' questions sensibly. If the nurses do not understand a research project, the parents are likely to complain that they are faced by a 'wall of silence', which may well reduce the likelihood of co-operation in the project. In particular nurses can help parents and children to understand what a research project will involve for them day to day. Research projects often require a number of procedures to be carried out over a period of time: it is not uncommon for parents not to realize this as they give consent, since it is unusual in the United Kingdom to use the sorts of consent form sometimes employed in the United States of America, which spell out all the procedures involved in a research project step by step.

Information for consent

Having informed other staff in the unit where the research is to take place and selected a suitable potential subject, the investigator must next seek to gain the consent of the parents or guardian of the child, and the assent of the child himself where appropriate: the latter requirement was inserted into the Helsinki Declaration when amended in 1983.[38] The word *must* is used quite deliberately: as was discussed in Chapter 6, voluntary and informed consent is mandatory to turn what would otherwise be a trespass and in some cases an assault into a legally sanctioned act. This point needs to be emphasized since the working group had evidence from several sources that some researchers in the United Kingdom do not inform parents that research procedures are being carried out on their children, and do not seek their consent. This evidence was of four sorts. First, many published papers made no mention of the gaining of parental consent for research on children, which does not necessarily, of course, mean that it was not obtained. Some examples, however, indicate that consent was unlikely to have been obtained; in the report[35] mentioned earlier of the use of a new colonoscope for proctosigmoidoscopy, it is difficult to suggest that the phrase 'without formality' means anything other than that no formal consent was obtained from the subjects' parents. Secondly, the working group received a copy of a proposal for research on neonates at a teaching hospital, which included the statement: 'It has not been the policy in the Special Care Baby Unit at . . . for informed consent to be obtained for this type of study.' (The particular study was a physiological one.) Thirdly, was the accumulated experience of the working group's own members. Fourthly, was the information provided by the survey of research ethics committee chairmen, which showed that one-sixth of such committees do not always insist on researchers gaining consent from the parents or guardian of a child, before that child may be entered into a research project.

That some paediatric investigators, with the approval of their research ethics committees, have dispensed with the obtaining of informed consent for research procedures is understandable in view of the very real difficulties that are faced. These are greatest in the field of neonatal medicine since procedures, to be of any value, often need to be started within a few hours, or even minutes, of birth. A recent study of the possible value of phenobarbitone in the prevention of periventricular haemorrhage in very low-birth-weight infants was carried out at the Hammersmith Hospital in West London;[39] the local research ethics committee required written parental consent before any infant could be entered into the trial. The consultant in charge of the trial described a typical occasion when consent was sought: 'a 17-year-old unmarried girl was transferred at 28 weeks gestation from Hertfordshire bleeding vaginally and was delivered by Caesarian section at Hammersmith. As the mother came round from the general anaesthetic, a paediatrician introduced himself to her and told her that she had a tiny baby weighing just 2 lbs and having breathing difficulties. Having explained that the baby was being kept alive by a mechanical ventilator, the paediatrician then went on to tell her that the baby had a 50% chance of having a brain haemorrhage and that a minority of such babies survived with longterm handicap, such as spastic cerebral palsy. He continued to tell her that a drug called phenobarbitone, used in epilepsy, might reduce the chances of brain haemorrhage and that he wished to put her baby into a trial in which nobody would know whether her baby was receiving phenobarbitone or salt water. This information was being imparted to a partly sedated 17-year-old who had never had anything to do with premature babies, never heard of babies getting brain haemorrhages, had never heard of phenobarbitone but had heard that the word 'spastic' was used as a form of abuse for clumsy idiots. Because treatment had to be started within four hours of birth, it was not possible to delay the explanation.' (A. Whitelaw, personal communication.)

The consultant summed up his experience in the trial thus: 'informed parental consent in this trial has caused excessive anxiety to parents, has occupied much highly skilled time and has achieved very little enlightenment'. Such comments are fairly typical of many investigators in neonatal research and need to be considered. Parental anxiety is an extremely common condition on special care baby units: in the case of this 17-year-old Hertfordshire girl, it would be impossible to distinguish how much of her anxiety was caused by some degree of understanding of the condition of her baby and how much was caused by the idea of an experiment being performed on that baby. The alternative, practised elsewhere, would be to give the mother no information and simply to get on with the research. When, a few days later, she discovers that her baby has been used for research, will her anxiety be any the less? This appears to be a situation in which it would be wise to apply the Golden Rule: how many neonatologists would be happy for their own infants to be in special care baby units other than those in which they normally work, knowing that they (the neonatologists) would not be asked for their consent to any research that the other units might wish to carry out?

The second comment concerned the amount of time that the process of obtaining consent took up. This seems to be inevitable if a serious attempt to inform the parents is to be made. The third comment was to the effect that very little enlightenment resulted from the process. This need not always be the case: what is being presented is the old problem of how to achieve better communication between doctor and patient or parent. There are well-recognized ways of improving communications, but many doctors do not appreciate just how simple they must keep the level of language that they use. The use of written information also helps communication. There have been occasional reports to show just how successful attempts at informing potential research subjects can be. Woodward reported[40] on attempts to inform volunteer subjects in cholera research about the nature of cholera; he then set a multiple choice examination both for the potential subjects and various groups of medically-trained personnel. The volunteers gained higher marks than any of the medical groups, even outscoring some tropical medicine experts. They were not a particularly well-educated group, and had received explanations of cholera interspersed over 1 to 2 days with having a medical history taken, being examined and having psychological tests.

The working group considered at length whether there were occasions when investigators would be justified in dispensing with parental consent. It concluded that the occasions on which an investigator would so be justified were extremely rare. It recognized that the requirement for consent might sometimes make a research project much more difficult to carry out, but was concerned that investigators should not develop an inflated sense of the importance of their research in comparison with their duties to protect the autonomy both of child subjects and their parents. In discussing consent in emergencies, Wilkinson, a former professor of paediatric surgery, says in the *Dictionary of medical ethics*:[41] 'When such consent cannot be obtained treatment should be confined to the minimum necessary to deal with the emergency.' If, on one of the rare occasions the research is so important that a research ethics committee allows the investigators to proceed without consent, it is important that the investigators should explain to the parents as soon as possible afterwards what has happened: there is no justification for continued concealment.

There is one other sort of research in which there may be an ethical justification not to inform parents, although it is doubtful whether that would make it legally acceptable, namely psychological research in which awareness of the hypothesis would alter the behaviour of the respondent so as to make the hypothesis untestable. If one wished to examine the effects on children of having quarrelling parents, one might either give a potential research family full information, in which case it would either refuse to take part or else would co-operate but greatly modify its behaviour, or one might give less precise information, representing the project as part of a larger investigation of family relationships. This could be an important area of research, since it is known that some children seem to be relatively unaffected by family disturbance: but it is not known which children or why. Various opinions were given by members of the working group about the ethics of such a proposal. One member thought it illustrated the fundamental cleavage between the good of society and the interests of the individuals, and would have been unhappy in that instance to allow the interests of society to supercede the interests of the family. The question of whether informed consent required foreknowledge of the particular aims of a project was raised; it was thought that, usually, any disguising of the broad general nature of a project would mean that informed consent was not possible. One test of the information given was suggested: if a research subject would not still wish to participate in a research project if he were given more information about it, then the original consent was not fully informed. The doctrine of the economy of truth was also stated: that one is under an obligation to reveal all pertinent and truthful information but one is under no similar obligation to reveal unnecessarily that which would disrupt a worthwhile relationship. The ethical problems raised by the use of deception in research are discussed thoroughly by Diener and Crandall.[42]

It remains the general rule that valid consent depends on full information; it also remains a general rule that it is impossible to define what is meant by full information. Burnham[43] provided a splendid parody of American consent forms in demonstrating the information needed for consent to repair a hernia. His consent form ends after two pages with the statement: 'I understand the anatomy of the body, the pathology of the development of hernia, the surgical technique that will be used to repair the hernia, the physiology of wound healing, the dietetic chemistry of the foods that I must eat to cause healing, the chemistry of body repair, and the course which my physician will take in treating any of the complications that can occur as a sequel of repairing an otherwise simple hernia'; and space is provided for the signatures of the patient, lawyer for the patient, lawyer for the doctor, lawyer for hospital, lawyer for anesthesiologist, mother-in-law, and a notary public. English law, however, retains a concept of the reasonable man, or 'the man on the Clapham omnibus'. It does not require doctors or researchers to go to excessive lengths in disclosing pertinent information; but it does require researchers and others to use the standards of accepted good practice in reaching their own judgement as to what information is necessary.

While the above provides only a general framework, it is possible to suggest one rather more specific rule: that investigators should always disclose what is actually going to be done to a research subject. It may be unreasonable to expect an investigator to specify all the possible risks of a procedure, although his local research ethics committee should consider all the possible risks and may advise him as to which risks he must disclose. There is some legal evidence to suggest, however, that full disclosure of physical procedures is needed. A court in Saskatchewan awarded a student substantial damages for injuries suffered during a research procedure,[44] on the grounds that he had not given a fully informed consent: he had consented to catheterization of his brachial artery, but had not been informed that the catheter would be advanced into his heart. Incomplete information may also have less obvious effects. A lady doctor returned to the hospital at which she had trained to give birth to her first child. Two hours after delivery of a normal infant she was asked by an investigator whether her infant could be used in a trial of a new thermometer that measured the temperature of the eardrum. She gave her consent and went to a laboratory to observe the procedure two hours later. When she arrived she found her infant totally immobilized and with an oesophageal thermometer in place. She had not been informed of the degree of restraint that would be needed, nor that a thermometer would be passed into the oesophagus: she had assumed that a thermometer in the rectum – a standard practice in infants – would be used for comparison. Her immediate feeling was of tremendous guilt for having failed to protect her child, a feeling which remained with her for years afterwards.

One possible solution to the various problems in giving suitable information to parents would be to have an information sheet printed, using a language level that is likely to be comprehended – various tests of readability are now available. Again, this is an area in which research ethics committees could provide a lead for investigators; at present only 11 per cent of the committees always insist on written information being given to parents, and half of them never so insist. The exercise of having to write explanations in simple language could prove of considerable benefit to those investigators who have hitherto thought their fields of research too complicated to explain to lay people: they are likely to find that it is almost always possible to make such explanations readily comprehensible. (The working group is well aware that a simpler level of language would be required than has been used in this report!) An additional benefit of writing explanations in simple language is that it would help the investigator to provide an explanation that older children could also understand. One difficulty with conventional single oral explanations is the small proportion of the information offered that is retained after the end of the interview. Cassileth *et al.*[45] provided one example of this: 'Within one day of signing consent forms for chemotherapy, radiation therapy or surgery, 200 cancer patients completed a test of their recall of the material in the consent explanation, and filled out a questionnaire regarding their opinions of its purpose, content and implications. Only 60% understood the purpose and nature of the procedure, and only 55% listed even one major risk or complication . . . Most patients believed that consent forms were means to protect the physician's rights.' On the other hand,

Woodward's example,[40] discussed earlier, showed that volunteers in cholera research could be very well informed and could retain the information for three months.

Although the working group was not aware of any studies of the use of written information, there appear to be good reasons for suggesting that it may be of benefit to many parents and their children. Another way of assisting parents to understand a project was mentioned earlier: ensuring that other staff in the unit understand the project, perhaps by using similar written information sheets. It is interesting that a report[46] of the use of parents' meetings, in two regional neonatal intensive care units, to increase support for parents, nowhere mentions research projects as having been discussed at any meetings: yet both units are known to have a considerable research output.

Consent

The two elements of consent that are vital were mentioned earlier: adequate information and voluntariness. Some of the difficulties in providing adequate information have been discussed; the difficulties in ensuring voluntariness tend to be rather more subtle. In fact, as a general rule, one can only trust investigators not to apply any coercion: it is indeed virtually unheard of for an investigator to be accused of trying to coerce someone into becoming a research subject. There are, however, some general measures that could be applied to ensure that consent is not only freely given, but seen to be freely given.

One form of persuasion, i.e payment for participation, has already been considered. Another form may be the demand that a decision be made straight away, generally for the pragmatic reason that the researcher is busy. Two-thirds of research ethics committees never insist that there should be any length of time between parents being given an explanation and being asked to give consent. Yet the provision of a period of time for reflection by parents would greatly assist them in coming to a freely given decision with which both parents were happy. The occasions when the research procedure needs to be performed urgently in order to be of any value are quite a small minority.

It may well be that investigators should be encouraged to take more responsibility for giving information and obtaining consent. The survey of research ethics committees showed that not only do several of them allow other doctors or nurses to give explanations to parents, but almost half the committees allow other doctors to obtain consent from the parents. Zerubavel[47] studied these processes in an American hospital and came to two pertinent conclusions. He developed the concept of 'floating responsibility', because it was observed that no one person was normally responsible for obtaining consent or for providing the information necessary for it. Essentially 'floating responsibility' describes the common occurrence that if a job is left to two or more people to do, without specifying that one of them should do it, it will not be done at all. He was also concerned about the impersonal way in which consent forms, that included information necessary for consent, were used. He thought that it was all too easy for those who presented the forms to patients to be effectively dissociated from them, and to provide no personal input of information.

There are therefore good reasons for suggesting that:

(i) Information should be given to the parents of a potential research subject by the investigator himself, and opportunities provided for discussion.

(ii) This should be backed up by an information sheet, written in simple language, which the parents can keep.

(iii) There should in general be a gap of at least one day between the giving of information and the requesting of consent.

(iv) The request for consent should be made by the investigator himself.

This procedure is suggested as being the most likely to obtain a free and informed consent; it is not intended to cover every possible situation. Similar constraints should be applied when assent is to be obtained from older children.

Child advocacy

It was suggested to the working group that there are some research projects in which it would be valuable to have a third party involved in the discussions between investigator and parents. Such a third party has been variously called 'the patient's friend', a 'guardian of the child's interests,' or a 'child advocate': the last expression will be used in this discussion.

Recommendation 7 of the US National Commission's report *Research involving children*[48] suggests the provisions that an Institutional Review Board should make to ensure that a child's assent and a parent's consent are properly solicited. It does not specify the need for a child advocate, but later discussion of the recommendation suggests that a child advocate may sometimes be needed. When, however, the final regulations for protecting children involved as research subjects in the United States were published in March 1983, they included no general recommendation for the involvement of a child advocate. The only exception was that a child advocate should be appointed by an IRB whenever a ward of the state might become a research subject: in those circumstances the child advocate would act instead of a parent and could give or withhold consent.

The working group considered the involvement of a child advocate in research on children and decided that it could not recommend such involvement. It was felt that the presence of a child advocate would hinder the development of a proper working relationship between parents and child and the investigator, by reducing the trust of the parents in the investigator, and by reducing the personal responsibility perceived by the investigator for the parents and child. It is nevertheless worth rehearsing the arguments for and against the involvement of a child advocate.

The basic reason for recommending that a child advocate be involved lies in a recognition of the conflict of interest that exists between the doctor as investigator and the doctor as personal physician, and which has been discussed elsewhere. It is then possible to describe a number of purposes for a child advocate:

(a) To ensure that research approved by research ethics committees is carried out ethically and that no unapproved research procedures are performed.

(b) To provide information to parents and children about the nature of a research project and its risks and potential benefits, independently of the investigator.

(c) To advise researchers in the selection of children as research subjects so as to avoid the imposition of unnecessary risks on children already greatly at risk, and to advise on the competence of children to give or withhold assent.

(d) To ensure that any consent or assent given is voluntary and informed, and that parents are aware that they may withdraw their child from a project at any time.

The problems with such a role for a child advocate are considerable, not least because of the danger that the role will become adversarial. A description of the role of a patient advocate in adult research in the United States[50] tends rather to emphasize the information-gathering role of the advocate. While the advocate does monitor all requests for consent, he also acts as a channel for any queries or worries of the research subjects, follows up subjects to invite comment on the quality of their care during a project, oversees recruitment of volunteers, writes reports to the IRB, and reviews all payments to volunteers. Many of these duties are ones which would in the United Kingdom be regarded as the responsibility of the investigator: their performance by an advocate would tend to diminish trust between subjects and investigators. This diminution of trust is perhaps the principal objection to the idea of a child advocate, but there are some practical objections also:

(a) The advocate would be unlikely to have the necessary technical expertise to understand completely and to advise knowledgeably on the research; if he were knowledgeable, that knowledge would suggest undue affinity with the investigator.

(b) The advocate could only discourage parents from giving consent, and not persuade unwilling parents, so that it would take longer to recruit subjects.

(c) It remains unclear what sort of persons could act as advocates, by whom they would be appointed, whether they would be paid, and how their work could be arranged such that they would always be available when needed.

It seemed to the working group that these disadvantages and difficulties of having a child advocate outweighed the possible benefits to child subjects.

The actual procedure

It is perhaps superfluous to comment that all procedures must be carried out with the greatest possible care and skill by the re-searchers. It is not uncommon, however, for investigators to be carrying out relatively complicated procedures for the first time on children during a research procedure. It is incumbent upon them to use every possible opportunity to learn the procedure other than on children before using it on children.

Another comment on carrying out research procedures that is perhaps required by common sense is that whenever possible parents should be present. Put the other way round, this suggests that investigators should, if possible, try to perform procedures when parents are present, even if, for instance, it means having to do so in the late afternoon or evening when parents are most likely to visit. While all the influences on parental bonding with neonates remain to be elucidated, it is also important that parents be present when neonatal research procedures are being carried out. It should also be remembered that it is possible for older children to enjoy being involved in research procedures. Bartholome[51] commented that in discussions with children about clinical research proposals, many of them suggested that projects should be designed so that children would actually enjoy the experience. 'How ethically important is fun?'

Afterwards

The responsibility of an investigator to his subjects, or to the parents of his subjects, does not end as soon as he successfully completes the research procedure(s). If the project has involved only partial disclosure of intent, such as in observational psychological studies, for which fully informed consent was not obtained, then it is vital for the researcher to discuss the research fully with parents and subjects afterwards. The paper outlining unexpected emotional and social effects in a diabetic study,[52] discussed more fully in Chapter 5, made the point that time should always be built into a project for discussion with, and support of, the subjects and their families. This seems to be a valuable general point, and the need for such discussion time probably increases with the complexity of the research project.

The final responsibility of the investigator is a more general one: he has a duty, not only to his subjects and to possible future bene-ficiaries of his research results, but also to the scientific community as a whole, to record and report his results accurately and honestly, both in the child's medical records and in the medical literature. It seems strange that it should be necessary to make the point, but a variety of episodes of dishonesty in science have been recorded in recent years. Whether the investigator be of the eminence of Sir Cyril Burt, or a student wanting to reduce the time spent on class work, the falsifying of results is equally unacceptable, and, by misleading future workers, may be positively dangerous. There is a further problem related to the reporting of results: research which was poorly conducted or produced no worthwhile results is much less likely to be reported than successful research. An adverse consequence that may therefore arise is that other investigators will attempt the same research, putting more children at risk, when in fact it is already known – but not generally known – that that research will fail. Perhaps there should be a *Journal of Pseudocyetic Research* in which failures or insignificant results could be recorded briefly to deter other investigators from repetition.

References

1. British Paediatric Association. Report of the Academic Board 1981-82: Research in Paediatrics. *Archs Dis. Childh.* **57**, 798 (1982).
2. *The medical research directory*. John Wiley, Chichester (1983).
3. Harpin, V.A. and Rutter, N. Making heel pricks less painful. *Archs Dis. Childh.* **58**, 226–8 (1983).
4. Drummond, M.F. and Stoddart, G.L. Economic analysis and clinical trials. *Controlled Clinical Trials* **5**, 115–28 (1984).
5. Morton, R.E. and Lawande, R. The diagnosis of urinary tract infection: comparison of urine culture from suprapubic aspiration and midstream collection in a children's out-patient department in Nigeria. *Ann. trop. Paediat.* **2**, 109–12 (1982).
6. Editorial. Secret randomised clinical trials. *Lancet* **ii**, 78–9 (1982).
7. Brewin, T.B. Consent to randomised treatment. *Lancet* **ii**, 919–21 (1982).
8. Hofmann, F. Misuse of randomized clinical trials. *Man and Medicine* **4**, 138–42 (1979).
9. Pugh, R.N.H. and Teesdale, C.H. Single dose oral treatment in urinary schistosomiasis: a double blind trial. *Br. med. J.* **286**, 429–32 (1983).
10. McMahon, J.E. A note on drug trials in schistosomiasis. *Trans. R. Soc. trop. Med. & Hyg.* **75**, 597–8 (1981).
11. Schafer, A. The ethics of the randomized clinical trial. *New Eng. J. Med.* **307**, 719–24 (1982).

12. Lockwood, M. Sins of omission? The non-treatment of controls in clinical trials: I. *Proc. Aristotelian Soc.* Suppl. **LVII**, 207–22 (1983).
13. Clayton, D.G. Ethically optimised designs. *Br. J. clin. Pharmac.* **13**, 469–80 (1982).
14. Altman, D.G. Statistics and ethics in medical research. In *Statistics in practice* (eds. S.M. Gore and D.G. Altman) pp.1-24. British Medical Association, London (1982).
15. Zelen, M. A new design for randomized clinical trials. *New Engl. J. Med.* **300**, 1242–5 (1979).
16. Burkhardt, R. and Kienle, G. Controlled clinical trials and medical ethics. *Lancet* **ii**, 1356–9 (1978).
17. Giertz, G. Ethics of randomised clinical trials. *J.med. Ethics* **6**, 55–7 (1980).
18. Tygstrup, N. Principles and problems of clinical trials: a European view. *Triangle* **19**, 93–6 (1980).
19. Vere, D. Controlled clinical trials: the current ethical debate. *J. R. Soc. Med.* **74**, 85–7 (1981).
20. Brook, I. Clindamycin in treatment of chronic recurrent suppurative otitis media in children. *J. Laryngol. Otol.* **94**, 607-615 (1980).
21. *British National Formulary No. 7.* British Medical Association and The Pharmaceutical Society of Great Britain, London (1984).
22. Forfar, J.O. and Arneil, G.C. (eds.) *Textbook of paediatrics* (3rd edn). p.2020. Churchill Livingstone, Edinburgh (1984).
23. DeBakey, L. Ethically questionable data: publish or reject? *Clin. Res.* **22**, 113–21 (1974).
24. Goel, K.M., Shanks, R.A., McAllister, T.A., and Follett, E.A.C. Prevalence of intestinal parasitic infestation, salmonellosis, brucellosis, tuberculosis, and hepatitis B among immigrant children in Glasgow. *Br. med. J.* **i**, 676–79 (1977).
25. Inner London Education Authority. *Policy on external research applications.* ILEA, London (1982).
26. Bodkin, C.M., Pigott, T.J., and Mann, J.R. Financial burden of childhood cancer. *Br. med. J.* **284**, 1542–4 (1982).
27. Smith, M.A. and Baum, J.D. Costs of visiting babies in special care baby units. *Archs Dis. Childh.* **58**, 56–9 (1983).
28. Mead, M. Research with human beings: a model derived from anthropological field practice. In *Experimentation with human subjects* (ed. P.A. Freund) pp.152–77. George Allen & Unwin, London (1972).
29. Beecher, H.K. Ethics and clinical research. *New Engl. J. Med.* **274**, 1354–60 (1966).
30. Pappworth, M.H. *Human guinea pigs.* Routledge & Kegan Paul, London (1967).
31. Durham, M. Pregnant women 'at risk' in research tests. *The Observer (London)* 6th Nov., p.4, col. 1–4 (1983).
32. Aggett, P.J. and Taylor, F. A normal paediatric amylase range. *Archs Dis. Childh.* **55**, 236–8 (1980).
33. Allen, P.A. and Waters, W.E. Development of an ethical committee

and its effect on research design. *Lancet* i, 1233–6 (1982).

34. Williams, C.B., Laage, N.J., Campbell, C.A., Douglas, J.R., Walker-Smith, J.A., Booth, I.W., and Harries, J.T. Total colonoscopy in children. *Archs Dis. Childh.* **57**, 49–53 (1982).

35. Nazer, H., Walker-Smith, J.A., Davidson, K., and Williams, C.B. Outpatient paediatric proctosigmoidoscopy: possible and useful. *Br. med. J.* **286**, 352 (1983).

36. Levene, M.I., Whitelaw, A., Dubowitz, V., Bydder, G.M., Steiner, R.E., Randell, C.P., and Young, I.R. Nuclear magnetic resonance imaging of the brain in children. *Br. med. J.* **285**, 774–6 (1982).

37. Congenital Disabilities (Civil Liability) Act 1976.

38. World Medical Association. *Declaration of Helsinki.* Recommendations guiding physicians in biomedical research involving human subjects. (Adopted, Helsinki, 1964; amended, Tokyo, 1975 and Venice, 1983.)

39. Whitelaw, A., Placzek, M., Dubowitz, L., Lary, S., and Levene, M. Phenobarbitone for prevention of periventricular haemorrhage in very low birth-weight infants. *Lancet* ii, 1168–70 (1983).

40. Woodward, W.E. Informed consent of volunteers: a direct measurement of comprehension and retention of information. *Clin. Res.* **27**, 248–52 (1979).

41. Wilkinson, A.W. Consent. In *Dictionary of medical ethics* (eds. A.S. Duncan, G.R. Dunstan, and R.B. Welbourn) (2nd edn) pp.113–17. Darton, Longman, & Todd, London (1981).

42. Diener, E. and Crandall, R. *Ethics in social and behavioral research,* pp.72–97. University of Chicago Press, Chicago (1978).

43. Burnham, P.J. Medical experimentation on humans. *Science* **152**, 448–50 (1966).

44. *Halushka* v. *University of Saskatchewan* 52 WWR 608 (1965).

45. Cassileth, B.R., Zupkis, R.V., Sutton-Smith, K., and March, V. Informed consent: why are its goals imperfectly realized? *New Engl. J. Med.* **302**, 896–8 (1980).

46. Dammers, J. and Harpin, V. Parents' meetings in two neonatal units: a way of increasing support for parents. *Br. med. J.* **285**, 863–5 (1982).

47. Zerubavel, E. The bureaucratization of responsibility: the case of informed consent. *Bull. Am. Acad. Psychiatry & the Law* **8**, 161–7 (1980).

48. National Commission for the Protection of Human Subjects of Biomedical and Behavioral Research. *Research involving children: Report and recommendations.* DHEW, 77-0004, Washington D.C. (1977).

49. Department of Health and Human Services. Additional protections for children involved as subjects in research (45CFR46). *Federal Register* **48**, 9814–20 (1983).

50. McGrath, K. and Briscoe, R.J. The role of the subject advocate in a community-based medical research facility. *IRB: a review of human subjects research* **3**(2), 6–7 (1981).

51. Bartholome, W.G. Ordinary risks of childhood (letter). *Hastings Center Report* **7**(2), 4 (1977).

52. Kinmonth, A.L., Lindsay, M.K.M., and Baum, J.D. Social and emotional complications in a clinical trial among adolescents with diabetes mellitus. *Br. med. J.* **286,** 952–4 (1983).

10

Summary and conclusions

Our working group on the ethics of clinical research on children was established because of the evident discrepancy between various extant guidelines on the conduct of such research. This discrepancy not only involves the legal and ethical bases of the guidelines, but also leads to practical difficulties. Our report has therefore attempted both to illuminate the ethical and legal frameworks within which research on children must be conducted, and to consider, in some depth, selected aspects of research common to many research projects involving children. In this chapter, after some general conclusions have been stated, our specific conclusions and recommendations are drawn together as they apply to the three principal groups of participants – parents and children, investigators, and research ethics committees.

General conclusions

Given the scientific and experimental basis of modern medicine, research on children is desirable and necessary in order to promote the health and well-being of children. Such research should take place only when an alternative such as *in vitro* research, or research on animals or adults, is not possible. (Chapter 3.)

> **We recommend** that research requiring children as subjects should not be undertaken unless there is a specific and demonstrable need to perform the research on children, and no other route to the relevant knowledge is available.

In all research on children, the general conventions for the conduct of research on human subjects – as given, for instance, in the Helsinki Declaration or the Proposed International Guidelines

(pp.14–15) – should apply:
i.e.

(a) the research must be scientifically sound with an identifiable prospect of benefit;
(b) the subjects must be selected equitably;
(c) risks to the subjects, and the number of subjects involved, must both be minimized;
(d) voluntary informed consent must be obtained from all subjects – or from their proxies – before any research procedure is started;
(e) subjects must be allowed to withdraw from a project at any time, and they and their parents should be assured that such withdrawal will not prejudice their ordinary treatment, if they are receiving any;
(f) subjects must be removed from a project as soon as there is any indication of possible harm, whether physical or psychological, being done to them as a consequence of their being research subjects;
(g) the privacy of subjects, and the confidentiality of data about them, must be protected;
(h) results must be written up honestly and accurately.

It is evident that an analysis of the risks and benefits of a proposed research project is a necessary part both of the scientific and of the ethical assessment of the project. Until now such analyses have tended largely to be intuitive. We have shown that several research risks can now be quantified, and that more could be if investigators and clinicians were to record accurately both the adverse events associated with particular procedures and the frequency of their occurrence. Similarly the developing use of various health indicators holds the prospect that some quantification of the potential benefits of a research project may be possible. (Chapter 5.)

We recommend that further efforts be made to develop scales quantifying risk and benefit, so as to reduce reliance on the qualitative descriptions of risk in use at present.

Until such time as quantitative scales of risk and benefit are in general use, however, the qualitative scale of risk used in the United States seems to be less confusing, although more unwieldy, than the scale used in the British Paediatric Association guidelines. The American scale employs the terms *'minimal'*, *'minor increase over minimal'*, and *'greater than minor increase over minimal';* quantitative equivalents of these descriptions of risk were suggested in Chapter 5.

The difficulties in defining completely the terms 'therapeutic research' and 'non-therapeutic research' have been discussed at length. In most cases, however, it will be possible to determine into which category a research *procedure* falls. The working group believes that, both legally and ethically, non-therapeutic research procedures on children are more difficult to justify than therapeutic research procedures. (Chapter 2.)

We recommend that non-therapeutic research procedures should not be carried out, if they involve greater than minimal risk to any individual child subject.

Examples have been given of the sorts of experiments that may be classified as innovative therapy. It is evident that some innovative therapies may expose children to high levels of risk. The working group believes it to be important that a doctor trying out an innovative therapy should cease to do so haphazardly as early as possible, by testing the therapy in a formal research programme if it shows any promise. (Chapters 2 and 9).

We recommend that there should be a limit on the number of times that an innovative therapy may be used on children, without its being submitted as a formal research project to a research ethics committee.

The working group is concerned at the possibility that similar research might be conducted at the same time by different research teams and that failed – and therefore unpublished – research might be repeated. It recognizes, of course, that in some cases repetition is desirable in order to check important results. It approves, however, the efforts of the British Paediatric Association to establish a register of current paediatric research in the United Kingdom, and hopes that investigators will use such a register to avoid unnecessary duplication.

The remainder of the recommendations and conclusions of the working group have been divided into sections entitled 'Parents and children', 'Investigators', and 'Research ethics committees'. The comments in each section will apply principally to those named, but will of course be relevant to a greater or less extent to all who are involved with research on children.

Parents and children

The duties of parents to their children have been discussed in Chapter 6, in which it was noted that in recent years courts have tended to apply a test of whether an activity was 'not against the interests' of a child rather than being 'in the best interests' of the child. The working group found it generally unhelpful to talk in terms of the 'rights' of parents.

We recommend that parents and guardians should be considered as trustees of a child's interests, rather than as having rights over the child. The prime consideration in any research involving children should be that it be not against the interest of any individual child.

We examined both the legal and ethical bases of the giving of proxy consent by parents or guardians for a research procedure on their child. We believe that such proxy consent for a therapeutic research procedure is in general legally valid and ethically acceptable. In the case of a non-therapeutic research procedure, however, there are strict limitations to that for which a proxy consent may be valid. (Chapter 6.)

We conclude that proxy consent by parents or guardians to a non-therapeutic research procedure on their child is legally valid and ethically acceptable only when the risk of such research to the child subject is no more than minimal.

The working group noted that various ages have been suggested as being that at which a child's assent or consent to a research procedure should be sought. Both the law and a knowledge of child development suggest that competence in understanding rather than a chronological age should determine a child's ability to give consent. There is, however, prima-facie evidence that a large majority of children aged 14 or over have the necessary competence to give or refuse consent, and that children aged 7 or over understand enough to be able to give or refuse assent. The working group discussed the relative importance to be given to a parent's or a guardian's giving or refusing of consent and that of the child, and made the following recommendations. It remains important, however, for each investigator to use his personal judgment as to how far he may carry out research procedures on a dissenting child subject, even though a parent or guardian has given consent. (Chapter 7.)

We recommend that:

(i) for consent to be valid on all (or any) interpretations of existing law, the consent of parent or guardian be required at all ages of the child; furthermore, the child's assent should be sought from the age of 7 upwards;

(ii) on a cautious view of the law, consent be deemed not to have been given if the parent or guardian of a child below 16 years refuses consent, *or* if a child over 14 years refuses consent;

(iii) notwithstanding the desirability of seeking the child's assent, for a child aged 7 to 14 years, the decision of parent or guardian to give consent for a therapeutic research procedure be deemed to override the refusal of assent by the child;

(iv) a non-therapeutic research procedure should not be carried out if a potential child subject aged 7 to 14 years refuses assent to it.

Investigators

'We are noted for being at once most adventurous in action and most reflective beforehand'. Pericles' description of the civilized democrats of Athens still provides a model that investigators would do well to follow, particularly in so far as they reflect beforehand on any research that they propose to carry out. The investigator should remember the words of the Helsinki Declaration: 'Concern for the interests of the subject must always prevail over the interests of science and Society.' The working group is convinced of the need for a wider group also to reflect on proposed paediatric research, regardless of whether the proposed procedures are extremely simple and of minimal risk or not. (Chapters 8 and 9.)

We recommend that all proposals for research on children be submitted to the appropriate research ethics committee for consideration.

The approval of the research ethics committee for a research project does not relieve the investigator of his ethical or legal responsibility for all interventions, and their effects, on the child subjects. The obligation of the investigator to the child subjects is primary, and the relationship between him and them is of the greatest importance to their welfare.

We recommend that investigators be encouraged to recognize that the research enterprise should be a partnership *with* the child subjects and their parents or guardians, rather than an activity undertaken *on* children.

Treating children as partners in research encourages investigators to regard each child subject as an individual, who may already be at greater or less risk physically, emotionally, or socially, than other child subjects in the project. (Chapters 5 and 9.)

We recommend that, in assessing the risks of a research project to an individual child subject, investigators take account not only of the risks of any proposed research procedures, but also of the cumulative medical, emotional, and social risks to which the child is already exposed or may become exposed, whether or not as a consequence of the research interventions.

It is important, both in the preparation and in the conduct of a research project, that the investigator allows sufficient time to recognise and protect the interests not only of the child subjects and their parents or guardians, but also of nursing and other staff who may be involved with them. Moreover, the scientific evaluation of research on children should take account of the emotional and behavioural outcomes for the subjects, in addition to the results of the research procedures. (Chapter 9.)

We recommend that investigators
  (i) devote sufficient time to explaining their projects to parents and child subjects, and to listening to the anxieties that will often arise;
 (ii) monitor whether the research procedures produce any emotional or behavioural disturbance in the child subjects;
(iii) deal promptly with any emotional or behavioural disturbance that does arise, either themselves or by appropriate referral;
(iv) devote sufficient time to explaining their projects to nurses and other staff involved with the child subjects and their parents, and to discussing any problems that may arise from the research procedures.

The need for parents to be allowed to stay with their children in hospital as much as they wish is now generally recognized, although unrestricted visiting is by no means universal. Just as it is important that treatment should not disrupt the relationship between child and parents, so it is that research procedures should not do so.

We recommend that research procedures on both neonates and older children should not be undertaken in such a way as to keep parent and child apart; where possible parents should be encouraged to be present.

We recommend that no financial or other inducements should be offered to parents or guardians to persuade them to enter their children into a research project; that any expenses incurred by parents or children by reason of participation in the research project should be paid, and that small gifts given to child subjects after completion of a research project should be allowed.

Research ethics committees: recommendations and draft rules

The survey of research ethics committees undertaken by the working group illustrates the large variations in structure and functioning of such committees. The working group recognizes that differing local circumstances will require certain differences in the committees serving those localities. As a way of summarizing our recommendations, we offer the following draft rules for research ethics committees. These could apply, prima facie, to all such committees, in so far as proposals for research on children may come before them. On those occasions, at least, competent paediatric advice should be available to each committee. See also IV and X below.

   I. *Objective:* the committee exists to maintain high ethical standards in the conduct of any clinical research procedure undertaken on human subjects by a particular – and defined – group of researchers, and to ensure that such research procedures do not endanger the safety or well-being of the subjects, or undermine public confidence in the conduct of medical research.

  II. *Accountability:* the committee is accountable, for meeting its objective, to the District Health Authority, Special Health Authority, or Board of Governors, as appropriate.

III. *Membership:* the committee shall consist of not fewer than five members and not more than twelve members. There shall be, at least, one member who is a local general practitioner, one member who is a nurse and one member whose profession is not in health care and who holds no position of employment by the body to whom the committee is accountable. In teaching hospitals and other large research centres there shall be a junior investigator (i.e. of registrar or senior registrar status) as a member of the committee. Ideally, the nursing member or members shall be involved directly in patient care rather than in administration.

A typical committee would be:

4 hospital doctors, 2 of whom at least should be involved in research work

at least 1 general practitioner

at least 1 ward sister

at least 2 members whose professions are not in health care

1 junior investigator

So far as is possible, members will be invited to serve on the committee in their personal capacities, rather than in respect of some office they hold. In order to function effectively, the committee must be able to work together as a body rather than as potential adversaries.

Opportunities will be provided for new members to be inducted into the role of the committee; new members will also be provided with copies of its constitution and of recognized guidelines for the conduct of research.

The names of committee members will be available to the body to whom the committee is accountable, and, on enquiry, to other persons with a legitimate interest.

IV. *Co-opted members:* the committee should co-opt specialists as required. When proposals are considered that involve children, the mentally ill or the mentally handicapped, there must be present at least one person expert in the care of the relevant group. The committee shall always have access to the expert advice of a statistician, since it would be unethical to approve statistically inept proposals.

V. *The chairman:* it is, in general, appropriate that the chairman be a hospital doctor working in the principal hospital or research centre of the area served. He will then be more readily available for the informal discussion with investigators that should be encouraged both in the planning and in the execution of research projects.

VI. *Length of service:* since there appears to be a long learning period for new members, it seems undesirable to set a limit to a member's length of service. If such a limit is thought to be necessary it should not be less than three years.

VII. *Quorum:* a quorum for a meeting of the committee shall be at least 50 per cent of its membership, including at least one member whose profession is not in health care.

VIII. *Conduct of business:*

(a) The committee shall have a standard application form on which each research proposal is submitted so as to ensure that all necessary and relevant information is provided. (See Appendix B.)

(b) There will be a contractual obligation on all employees of the relevant Health Authority to submit all proposals for research on human subjects to the committee.

(c) If a proposal does not include any invasive procedures and involves no more than minimal risk, the chairman shall be empowered to give his considered approval, if he thinks fit, without waiting for the next meeting of the committee. Any such authorization shall be open to discussion by the whole committee, but not to revocation.

(d) All proposals received by the chairman or secretary of the committee shall be circulated to all members of the committee at least one week before the meeting at which the proposals will be discussed.

(e) All proposals that cannot be approved under VIII(c) above will be considered at a meeting of the committee. Attempts will always be made to agree upon a decision, but if this proves impossible, a vote may be taken.

(f) The committee will conduct its business in such a way as to ensure the minimum delay in review of research proposals and will therefore meet as often as the rapid despatch of business requires. In exceptional circumstances it may conduct its business by post, but thorough discussion of submitted proposals should not be sacrificed in the interest of speedy decision.

(g) Since scientific validity is a pre-condition of ethical approval of any proposal for research, the committee must have assurance of this validity from persons competent to judge, particularly when, as commonly happens, the committee itself may not have this competence.

(h) The committee shall neither allocate funds for research, nor advise on their allocation.

IX. *Decisions and follow-up:*

(a) The committee may invite the principal investigator to meet it in order to provide clarification or further information on a research proposal.

(b) Decisions of the committee shall be communicated to the principal investigator in writing. They shall also be recorded in a committee minute book. Any substantive discussion of a proposal should also be recorded.

(c) If the committee decides that a proposal should be modified or rejected, it should be prepared to furnish the principal investigator, upon request, with reasons. In general however, the chairman, or another appropriate member of the committee, will discuss the committee's decision with the principal investigator.

(d) The work of the committee, to be successful, must depend on trust between the committee and the investigators it serves. The committee will investigate the progress and conduct of a research project only if it receives a complaint about that project. It may request progress reports from investigators, though it will recognize that it has no regulatory power over them.

(e) The committee will expect to be informed immediately of any adverse events occurring in an approved research project. Investigators are encouraged to approach the committee, or its chairman, at any time during the course of a project if either problems arise or a change in the original protocol becomes necessary.

X. *Research on children:* the committee will, in general, work to the following rules when considering proposals for research on children, and may apply them also to other sorts of research if appropriate.

1. The committee will wish to satisfy itself not only that a proposed research project on children is scientifically valid, but also that it holds out a possibility of substantial benefit to children. It will, in general, not be sufficient merely to show that the risk/benefit calculation is marginally favourable.

2. The committee will undertake its own assessment of the risks and benefits of a proposal. It may require the researcher to supply background information about the group of children from whom subjects will be chosen, so as to indicate whether they are likely already to be at risk emotionally or socially. In some circumstances, the committee may also wish to take account of the research record of the principal investigator. The investigator's obligation continually to assess the risk of proposed research procedures to each individual child subject is not diminished by the committee's duty to make a general assessment of the risks and benefits of the proposal for its own purposes.

3. The committee will normally require investigators themselves to explain a research project to the parents or guardians of potential child subjects. When the project involves greater than minimal risk to child subjects, the committee will also usually require investigators to provide a brief written explanation, in simple language

that the committee has approved. Such an explanation should include:

(a) a statement of the nature and purpose of the research project and procedures;

(b) a statement of any substantial risks and of potential benefits;

(c) a reminder of the parent's or guardian's right to withdraw the child from the project at any time;

(d) an invitation to ask questions;

(e) an invitation to stay with the child during research procedures, except when medically contraindicated: e.g. during surgical operations.

When the investigator does not speak the language of some or all of the child subjects or their parents, it will be particularly important to provide a written explanation in the appropriate language as well as to speak with the persons concerned through an interpreter.

4. The committee will encourage investigators to allow parents or guardians at least one day between the giving of an explanation and the giving of their consent to procedures of greater than minimal risk.

5. In the case of non-invasive research projects of minimal risk the committee will not usually require the consent of parents or guardians to be obtained in writing. The giving of oral consent should normally be witnessed, however, by someone who is not a member of the research team, and the fact of an explanation having been given and oral consent obtained should be recorded by the witness in the child's medical record.

6. For all other research projects the committee will require consent to be obtained in writing from the parents or guardians on a consent form approved by the committee.

7. In the case of any non-therapeutic research project the committee will require the investigator to obtain the

assent of any child subject aged 7 years or over, as well as parental consent, before he may proceed.

The intention of the working group in providing such draft rules for research ethics committees is not to make their approach unduly legalistic. The suggested rules are intended rather as a distillation of the conclusions of the working group on the evidence of good practice displayed in the responses of the chairmen of research ethics committees to the survey questionnaire (see Appendix A). The working group is certain that discussion of problems between investigators and research ethics committees is far more likely to promote the ethical conduct of clinical research than any rigid adherence to rules.

Appendix A

Questionnaire to chairmen of research ethics committees

This questionnaire is divided into six sections. Part of Section C, and Section D, need not be answered if your committee has considered no proposals for research on children in the past two years.

A. The committee

1. What group of researchers does the committee serve?
   (This might for instance be those in a hospital or a district, or the members of a Royal College.)
   Please specify: ....

2. (a) Within that group is it compulsory for all proposals for research on human subjects to be submitted to the committee?
   YES/NO
   (b) If it is compulsory to submit all research proposals, who made the rule?
   Please specify (if known): ....
   (c) If it is not compulsory to submit all research proposals, does the committee provide written guidance on the categories of research that should be submitted?
   YES/NO
   We should be very grateful to receive a copy of any such guidance.

3. How many members has your committee? ....

4. Of your committee how many members (including the chairman) are:
   (a) Paediatricians or paediatric sub-specialists ....

(b) General practitioners ....

(c) Others medically qualified, whether practising or not ....

(d) Nurses whether practising or not ....

(e) Others ....

5. What are the occupations or professions, most relevant to the work of the committee, of those members who are neither doctors nor nurses?
Please specify: ....

6. How many members of your committee have professional or expert experience of working with children (examples might be paediatric training, children's nursing, play (group) leadership, school teaching: please exclude all those whose experience is only of parenthood)? ....

7. How many members of your committee have particular experience in, or have made a special study of, ethical analysis or moral reasoning (for example, research, writing or teaching in medical ethics, theology, moral philosophy or the law; experience at the bar or in tribunals might also be relevant)? ...

8. What is the usual term of service of a committee member? (If unspecified, please enter an 'X') ....

9. Does your committee offer any briefing on its function to new members?
YES/NO
We should be very grateful to receive a copy of any briefing papers available.

10. Has there been any specific discussion in the committee, or in the group of researchers it serves, of the particular problems of research on children?
YES/NO
If YES, please give any further information available.

11. Does your committee allocate any funds for research?
YES/NO

B. Procedures

12. Does the committee consider separately the scientific merit of research proposals, when it is known that the researchers will seek funds from a grant-giving body?
YES/NO

13. Does the committee consider separately the scientific merit of research proposals, when there is no evidence that the researchers are seeking funds from grant-giving bodies?
YES/NO

14. If the answer to either or both of questions 12 and 13 is YES
    (a) Is the scientific review undertaken by:
        (i) A separate scientific review committee
        (ii) A sub-committee of the ethics committee
        (iii) Co-opted consultant
        (iv) Others
        If (iv) please specify: ....
    (b) When is the scientific review undertaken?
        Before ethical review
        During ethical review
        After ethical review

15. Does your committee encourage informal approaches by researchers prior to their submission of formal research proposals?
YES/NO

16. (a) Has your committee a standard application form for the submission of proposals for research on human subjects?
    YES/NO
    (b) Has your committee an application form specifically for the submission of proposals for research on children?
    (i.e. human beings from the moment of birth to their sixteenth birthday. 'Proposals for research on children' should include proposals in which some subjects will be adults and some will be children).
    YES/NO
We should be grateful to receive a copy of any such application forms.

17. Are research proposals normally circulated to each member of the committee?
YES/NO

18. How does your committee normally conduct its business?
    (a) By post
    (b) By meeting
    (c) By both the above
    (d) By other means
    If by other means, please specify: ....

19. How does your committee normally consider proposals for research on children?
    (a) By post
    (b) By meeting
    (c) By both the above
    (d) By other means
    If by other means, please specify: ....

20. Is approval for proposals for research on children ever given
    (a) By the chairman alone?
        YES/NO
    (b) By a sub-committee?
        YES/NO

21. How many times did the present committee, or the committee prior to April 1982 that served substantially the same group of researchers, meet?
    (a) in 1981
    (b) in 1982

22. On average, what percentage of the members of the committee attend its meetings?

C. Proposals for research on children

To answer the questions in this section precisely would, in most cases, require an unreasonable amount of work. For each question, therefore, unless precise figures are readily available, please give your estimate of the number, and tick the estimate box as appropriate.

23. (a) How many research proposals has your committee received in total in 1981 and 1982? ....
    (b) How many proposals for research on children has your committee received in 1981 and 1982? ....
If the answer to 23(b) is zero, please omit the rest of Section C, and only answer Section D if your committee has an agreed policy on the obtaining of consent to research on children.

24. Of the proposals for research on children, how many were:
    (a) Rejected outright ....
    (b) Modified substantially at the request of the committee .....
    (c) Modified slightly at the request of the committee ....
    (d) Approved unchanged ....
    (e) Withdrawn by applicants ....

25. Of the proposals for research on children that were rejected outright, how many were rejected for reasons of:
    (a) Poor research design
    (b) Acceptable research design but lack of scientific value
    (c) Ethical unacceptability
    (d) Inadequate arrangements for obtaining consent
    (e) Other problems
    If (e) please specify: ....

26. Of the proposals for research on children that were modified substantially or slightly, how many had problems of:
    (a) Poor research design ....
    (b) Acceptable research design but lack of scientific value ......
    (c) Ethical unacceptability ....
    (d) Inadequate arrangements for obtaining consent ....
    (e) Other problems ....
    If (e) please specify: ....

27. How much time elapses, on average, between the first submission of a proposal for research on children, and the committee's final decision on that proposal?
    Please state: ....

D. Consent to research on children

28. Does your committee insist that researchers gain consent from the parents or guardians of a child before that child may be entered into a research project?
    Always/Sometimes/Usually/Never

29. If consent is sought from parents or guardians, does your committee require them to be given a full explanation of the proposed research?
    Always/Sometimes/Usually/Never

30. Who usually gives the explanation to the parents or guardians?
    (a) The researcher
    (b) Another doctor
    (c) A ward sister
    (d) Any nurse
    (e) Other
    If (e) please specify: ....

31. Does the committee specify that a length of time should elapse between an explanation being given to parents or guardians,

and the request for their consent?
Always/Sometimes/Usually/Never

32. Whom does the committee allow to obtain consent from the parents?
   (a) The researcher
   (b) Another doctor
   (c) A ward sister
   (d) Any nurse
   (e) Other
   If (e) please specify: ....

33. Does the committee insist that consent to research on children be obtained from the parents or guardians in writing?
Always/Sometimes/Usually/Never

34. Does the committee require the obtaining of consent to research on children to be witnessed by a 'third party'?
Always/Sometimes/Usually/Never

35. Does the committee insist that parents or guardians of child research subjects be given a copy in writing of:
   (a) the explanation of the research?
      Always/Sometimes/Usually/Never
   (b) the consent form?
      Always/Sometimes/Usually/Never

36. From what age upwards, of a child research subject, does the committee require researchers to obtain the child's assent to a research procedure?
If no age is specified, please enter 'X' ....

37. From what age upwards, of a child research subject, does the committee consider the child's consent to be sufficient by itself for research procedures to be carried out?
If no age is specified, please enter 'X' ....

E. Follow-up

38. Does the committee ever require researchers to report back to it while a research project is in progress?
YES/NO

39. Does the committee ever require researchers to submit a final report on completion of a project?
YES/NO

40. Has the committee ever received complaints, about research on children that it had approved, from:
    (a) Doctors
    (b) Nurses and other health professionals
    (c) Parents
    (d) Community Health Council
    (e) Others
    (f) No complaints received
    If (e) please specify: ....

41. If any complaints about research on children have been received, were the complaints based on:
    (a) Misunderstanding
    (b) The lack of scientific value of the project
    (c) Poor research design
    (d) Ethical unacceptability
    (e) The emotional distress caused to the child
    (f) The physical risk to the child
    (g) Other reasons
    If (g) please specify: ....

42. Did the committee become aware, in 1981 and 1982, of any research projects carried out within its jurisdiction for which ethical approval had not been sought?
    YES/NO
    If YES, how many unapproved projects were discovered?

F. Guidelines

43. How useful has the committee found the following ethical statements in its discussions?
    (a) Medical Research Council Annual Report 1962–63 'Responsibility in investigations on human subjects'
    (b) Royal College of Physicians (1973): 'Supervision of the ethics of clinical research investigations in institutions'
    (c) DHSS Circular HSC (IS) 153 (1975): 'Supervision of the ethics of clinical research investigations and fetal research'
    (d) British Paediatric Association (1980): 'Guidelines to aid ethical committees considering research involving children'
    (e) World Medical Association (1975), 'The Helsinki declaration'.

Very Helpful/Helpful/Unhelpful/Chairman unaware of existence/Committee aware of existence, but had no discussion

44. If there are any proposals for research on children that have caused your committee particular difficulty, please give any details available here. They will of course be treated in the strictest confidence.

45. If there are any other matters concerned with the workings of your committee, of which you think that our Working Group should be aware, particularly as they may affect answers to previous questions, please mention them here: ....

46. Are there any changes in the structure and functions of research ethics committees that your committee would like to see?

47. If, when the responses to this questionnaire have been analysed, discussion of some activities of research ethics committees is needed in greater depth, would you be willing to talk to the research fellow?
YES/NO
If YES, please give name (in block letters)

48. Position, relative to the committee, of person completing questionnaire.

Reminder

Questions 2(c), 9, and 16 contain requests for documents that your committee may be able to provide. If any or all of the documents are available, please enclose them with this questionnaire in the reply-paid envelope provided.

Appendix B

Standard application form for ethical approval of research projects

In Chapter 8, p.169, it was suggested that research ethics committees would benefit from the use of standard application forms for ethical approval of research projects, since only a minority at present use such forms. The working group was sent several application forms that are in use and suggests the following example of a standard application form as being likely to elicit most of the information that a committee would routinely require.

APPLICATION TO RESEARCH ETHICS COMMITTEE FOR APPROVAL OF PROPOSED RESEARCH PROJECT

(N.B. The application should be made in simple and non-technical language, since it must be capable of being understood by the lay and nursing members of the committee.)

1. **Investigators.** (a) List names, qualifications, positions, departmental addresses, and functions in the proposed research of all investigators. (b) Name of principal investigator. (c) Experience of principal investigator in the field of research concerned.
2. **Place:** where research will be undertaken.
3. **Title of Project.**
4. **Objective of research:** i.e. state the hypothesis which is to be tested.
5. **Scientific background.** If similar work has been done anywhere previously, state why it needs to be repeated. If it has not been done before, has the problem been worked out as fully as

possible using animals or other alternative research methods?

6. **Design of the study.** State briefly what will actually be done, what measurements will be made, and how the results will be analysed. Has a statistician been consulted?

7. **Subjects.** Give details of method of recruitment, numbers, age groups for each category: patients, controls, healthy volunteers. Will those who are pregnant or involved in other research be excluded? Will any subjects be in a dependent position to the investigators? Will volunteers receive any payment?

8. **Informed consent.** How will consent be obtained from the subject, or the subject's parent or guardian? If in writing, please attach a copy of the form to be used. How much time will be allowed between giving an explanation of the research and requesting consent? Will consent be witnessed?

9. **Permission of other professionals.** Will subjects' general practitioners, or the consultants in overall charge of their cases, be asked for permission to enter the subjects into the study?

10. **Substances to be given:** i.e. drugs, special diets, isotopes, vaccines, etc. State route, dose, frequency, precautions. For isotopes, which radiation protection officer approved the dosage?

11. **Samples to be obtained:** i.e. blood, urine, cerebrospinal fluid, biopsy specimens, etc. State type of sample, frequency of sampling, amount of each sample.

12. **Other procedures.** Give details of any other procedures to be employed, e.g. X-rays, endoscopy, anaesthesia, cannulation, etc.

13. **Hazards.** Please specify possible discomfort, pain, limitation of activity, inconvenience, or expense likely to be incurred by patients.

14. **Risks.** What risks are involved in the study? State possible injuries to subjects and the probability of them occurring.

15. **Benefits.** Will the subjects receive any benefits from participation?

16. **Hospital facilities.** Will the project have any significant effect on the workload of nurses, laboratories, outpatient departments, etc.?

17. **Drugs.** What is the precise regulatory status of any drugs or appliances to be used – i.e. is there a product licence, a clinical

trials certificate or a clinical trials exemption? If the project is a drug trial sponsored or initiated by an industrial company, has the company provided a written statement accepting strict liability for any injuries to subjects?

18. **Investigators' interests.** Specify any financial or other direct benefit to investigators or their department arising from the study.

19. **Paediatric projects.** (a) If the study is not intended to benefit the child subjects, is the risk realistically judged to be minimal? (b) Will the assent of the child subjects be obtained?

Please supply, with this application, copies of:

   (i) any written explanation to be given to potential subjects;
  (ii) the proposed consent form;
 (iii) any poster or advertisement to be used to recruit volunteers;
 (iv) any written statement from an industrial company concerning its acceptance of liability for injuries to subjects;
  (v) the full protocol for the study, i.e. the relevant part of a grant application;
 (vi) any questionnaire to subjects that is to be used in the study.

Glossary

A fortiori: Even more so; with yet stronger reason.

Amylase: An enzyme (protein), produced by the pancreas, which assists the digestion of carbohydrates.

Anaphylaxis: An acute and severe reaction, sometimes fatal, to a substance to which a person is allergic.

Anorectal manometry: The measurement of pressure in the anus and rectum in various circumstances.

Anticoagulant: A substance that stops blood from clotting.

Audiometry: The testing of hearing.

Bacteraemia: The presence of bacteria in the bloodstream.

Bacteriuria: The presence of bacteria in the urine.

Brachial: Of the arm.

Bronchiolitis: An acute respiratory disorder of infancy.

Bronchospasm: Narrowing of the airways within the lungs, as in asthma.

Cannulation: The passage of a small tube through a hole, generally into a fluid-filled cavity such as the bladder or a blood-vessel.

Catheter: A flexible tube such as might be used for cannulation.

Cellulitis: Infection of the skin and tissues lying just beneath it.

Chemotherapy: Treatment of disease by chemicals; usually used to refer either to the treatment of cancers with cytotoxic drugs, or to the treatment of infections with antibiotics.

Colonoscope: Instrument, passed via the rectum, to inspect the colon visually.

Cytomegalovirus: A DNA virus, similar to herpes, which causes an illness like glandular fever in older children; infection of a fetus in the womb may lead to brain damage and problems with hearing and vision.

Cytotoxic: Cell-killing: used of drugs that kill cancer cells faster than normal cells.

Decibel: A measure of the loudness of sound using a logarithmic scale: 0 decibels (dB) is the threshold of hearing of a normal ear, 40 dB is a whisper, 80 dB a shout, 130 dB a jet engine a few feet away and 170 dB a large bore rifle shot – for about one thousandth of a second.

Deontological: The name given to ethical theories which seek the justification of acts or principles in conformity to duty, especially, in the context of this inquiry, the duty to respect rights.

Dura: The main membrane covering the brain and spinal cord.

Electrocardiogram: Record of electric currents generated by a person's heart beating.

Endoscope: Instrument for viewing internal parts of the body.

Enuresis: Involuntary urination.

Ex abundanti cautela: Taking the most cautious view.

Ex hypothesi: According to the hypothesis; it follows from what is said.

Fluorouracil: An antimetabolite cytotoxic drug, which interferes with the synthesis of DNA and RNA; used for treatment of solid tumours such as cancer of breast or colon.

Gastroscope: Instrument for viewing the stomach.

Gentamicin: An aminoglycoside antibiotic, very useful in a wide variety of infections, but has to be given by injection.

Giardia lamblia: A common protozoal parasite world wide, that causes chronic diarrhoea in children.

Glucose tolerance test: A test used in the diagnosis of diabetes.

Haemoglobin: An iron-containing substance in red blood cells that carries oxygen from the lungs to other tissues.

Haemolytic disease: Also known as Rhesus haemolytic disease or haemolytic disease of the newborn. A disease of infants, whose blood is incompatible with that of their mothers, resulting in severe jaundice and anaemia.

Hepatoblastoma: An embryonic malignant tumour of the liver.

Hirschsprung's disease: A congenital disorder of the nerve supply to the lower gut, resulting in severe constipation in affected children.

Histology: The study of the structure of tissues microscopically.

Hyaline membrane disease: A respiratory disorder, often severe, of premature babies, in which the fine structures of the lung are lined with a thick membrane and tend to collapse. Ventilatory assistance is frequently needed.

Hyperlipaemia: An abnormally high level of fats in the blood.

Hypertrophic pyloric stenosis: An abnormal thickening of the muscle surrounding the outlet from the stomach which blocks it: occurs a few weeks after birth.

Hypospadias: A developmental abnormality in which the urethra opens on the underside of the penis.

Hypotension: Abnormally low blood pressure.

Impedance tympanometry: Measurement of the pressure in the middle ear cavity and of the mobility of the eardrum.

Indian childhood cirrhosis: A degenerative disease of the liver most commonly occurring in Asian children in the first years of life.

In limine: At the outset.

Intracranial: Within the skull.

Intraperitoneal: Within the abdominal cavity.

Intrauterine: Within the womb.

Ketamine: An anaesthetic agent given by injection.

Laparotomy: A surgical incision through the abdominal wall.

Leishmaniasis: Infection caused by a protozoal parasite that may affect various organs of the body.

Lumbar puncture: The passage of a needle between two vertebrae in the lower back into the space surrounding the spinal cord – generally to obtain a sample of cerebrospinal fluid.

Lymphoma: Malignant tumour of the lymph nodes and spleen – often leading to an illness similar to leukaemia.

Malum in se: Wrong in itself.

Meconium: Contents of fetal lower intestine: forms first faeces of neonate.

Meningitis: Infection of the membranes surrounding the brain and spinal cord.

Meningococcus: A bacterium causing a very acute form of meningitis that may be epidemic in spread.

Micturition: The process of passing urine.

Nasogastric: Passing via the nose into the stomach.

Neural tube defects: Various congenital malformations of the skull and spinal cord: relatively common are spina bifida in which the vertebrae do not fuse normally around the spinal cord, and anencephaly in which much of the brain and skull is absent.

Neuroblastoma: A malignant tumour arising in tissue of the sympathetic nervous system.

Nuclear magnetic resonance: A method for defining the character of covalent bonds by measuring the magnetic moment of the atomic nuclei involved: the phenomenon has been harnessed to provide pictures similar to X-rays but which are more informative.

Oesophagus: The gullet, between the throat and the stomach.

Oncology: The study of tumours.

Osteomyelitis: Infection of a bone and/or bone marrow.

Percutaneous: Through the skin.

Periconceptional: Around the time of conception.

Perinatal: Around the time of birth; when used statistically, from end of 28th week of gestation to end of first week of life.

Peritonitis: Infection or inflammation of the membranes lining the abdominal cavity.

Periventricular haemorrhage: Bleeding into those parts of the brain surrounding the ventricles (fluid filled cavities in the brain).

Phenothiazine: One of a group of chemicals – 'major tranquillizers' – that are antipsychotic in action.

Placebo: Literally 'I shall please'. Substances that are pharmacologically inert but which may exert psychological effects.

Pneumothorax: The presence of air in the pleural cavity, between a lung and the chest wall, leading to partial or complete collapse of the lung.

Proctosigmoidoscopy: Instrumental examination of the rectum and lower part of the colon.

Pseudocyetic: Of a false pregnancy (i.e. when a woman or man is expanding as in pregnancy but is not pregnant).

Pseudomembranous colitis: Inflammation of the colon due to bacterial overgrowth with *Clostridium difficile,* usually an acute result of treatment with certain antibiotics.

Rectum: Lower part of large intestine ending at the anus.

Retrolental fibroplasia: Overgrowth of retinal blood-vessels leading to fibrosis in the posterior chamber of the eye, retinal detachment and blindness.

Rhabdomyosarcoma: A malignant tumour of muscle in young children (often 2 to 4 years old).

Rheumatic carditis: Inflammation of part or all of the heart in rheumatic fever.

Schistosomiasis: Bilharzia: a common parasitic disease of the tropics involving infestation by a fluke in the urinary or intestinal tracts; transmitted via fresh water snails.

Sensorineural deafness: Deafness, caused by damage to the inner ear, auditory nerve, or brain, that is almost always irreversible.

Septicaemia: The presence of infection (sepsis) in the bloodstream.

Shigellosis: Dysentery caused by Shigella bacteria.

Streptomycin: One of the earlier antibiotics to be developed: now used just in the treatment of tuberculosis.

Thalidomide: A sedative drug, withdrawn from use in the early 1960s when it was found to cause a high incidence of deformed fetuses in pregnant women, which has now found a strictly limited use in treating a skin disease.

Thrombophlebitis: Inflammation of a vein combined with some clotting of blood within the vein.

Thrombosis: A blood clot within a blood vessel.

Trypanosomiasis: A parasitic infection spread by flies: the American version is Chaga's disease, and the African is sleeping sickness spread by tsetse flies.

Tympanocentesis: Puncture of the ear drum in order to remove fluid from the middle ear cavity.

Ultrasonography: The process of detecting the reflections of very high frequency soundwaves in order to visualize the shape of body organs.

Uraemia: The presence of abnormally high levels of urea in the bloodstream – indicative of renal failure.

Ureter: The tube conveying urine from the kidney to the bladder.

Urethra: The tube that conveys urine from the bladder to the outside world.

Urticaria: An intensely itchy skin eruption characterized by weals.

Utilitarian: The name given to ethical theories which seek the justification of acts or principles in their consequences for good or the avoidance of harm. Since there are many such theories, it must not be assumed that objections to one of them serve to refute others.

Venepuncture: Puncture of a vein.

Venesection: Withdrawal of blood by puncture of a vein.

Water flux: The rate of flow of water from one part of the body to another.

Index

Asterisks indicate research projects discussed in the text.